Jung and Yoga

Marie-Louise von Franz, Honorary Patron

**Studies in Jungian Psychology
by Jungian Analysts**

Daryl Sharp, General Editor

JUNG AND YOGA

The Psyche-Body
Connection

JUDITH HARRIS

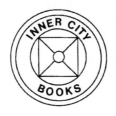

For Vanda Scaravelli (1908-1999),
my teachers—Esther Myers, Mary Stewart and Monica Voss—
and for my students and analysands, who, along with C. G. Jung, inspired this work.

In gratitude to: Mary Hamilton, Ethel Harris, Anne Maguire, René
Malamud, David Mandel, Paula Reeves, Andreas Schweizer,
Ann Skinner, Ursula Ulmer, Marion Woodman and Tony Woolfson.

Canadian Cataloguing in Publication Data

Judith Harris
    Jung and yoga: the psyche-body connection

(Studies in Jungian psychology by Jungian analysts; 94)

Includes bibliographical references and index.

ISBN 0-919123-95-3

1. Yoga—Psychological aspects.
2. Jungian psychology.
I. Title. II. Series.

BL1238.52.H37 2001   150.19'54   C00-931767-8

INNER CITY BOOKS
Box 1271, Station Q
Toronto, ON M4T 2P4, Canada

Telephone (416) 927-0355 / Fax (416) 924-1814
E-mail: icb@inforamp.net / Web site: www.innercitybooks.net

Honorary Patron: Marie-Louise von Franz.
Publisher and General Editor: Daryl Sharp.
Senior Editor: Victoria Cowan.

INNER CITY BOOKS was founded in 1980 to promote the
understanding and practical application of the work of C.G. Jung.

Cover: The ray of light of infinity (see below, page 112).

Printed and bound in Canada by University of Toronto Press Incorporated

CONTENTS

See final pages for descriptions of other Inner City Books

East and West
Can no longer be kept apart.
—Goethe.

Rabbi [Simha Bunam of Pzhysha] taught:
This is how we must interpret the first words in the scriptures:
"In the beginning of God's creation of the heaven and the earth."
For even now, the world is still in a state of creation.
When a craftsman makes a tool and it is finished,
it does not require him any longer.
Not so with the world!
Day after day, instant after instant,
the world requires the renewal of the powers of the
primordial world through which it was created,
and if the power of these powers were withdrawn from it
for a single moment, it would lapse into chaos.
—Martin Buber, *Tales of the Hasidim: The Early Masters.*

Foreword

In *Jung and Yoga: The Psyche-Body Connection,* Judith Harris goes to the heart of darkness to find the new light. As a young musician, she delighted in music pouring through her fingers as they danced with the piano keys. By the time she was twenty, however, she was forced to recognize that her own body had become an abject, traumatized instrument, no longer able to magnify the music that was attempting to come through her fingers. Faint glimmerings kept her in touch with the life force at her core: ballet lessons, yoga, desperate searching from healer to healer. These eased her physical pain and opened hope for a life that could be lived authentically. Interestingly, she knew that somewhere within her was a life waiting to be born.

Gradually, she became aware that her physical problems could not be resolved without attention to their psychic components. She entered Jungian analysis and coordinated her yoga practice with her analytic work. In that combination, her bodysoul work began and with it her journey into living with angels and demons. That matrix became the source of her present analytic practice and this book.

Jung and Yoga: The Psyche-Body Connection has a paradox at its core—a paradox that we all have to face if we undergo the initiation that takes us to the depths of our own creativity. Nietzsche states that paradox very naturally: The tree that grows to heaven must send its roots to hell. Obviously, a tree without roots will topple when a storm hits. But few of us live as if we believe it. Jung repeatedly warned people born in the West to ground their yoga practice in the body if they wished to dare the heights of spiritual insight. In the East, the Indian world in which yoga was born is firmly rooted in the soil of the matriarchal mother. Western culture is not; its mother *(mater)* is materialism—money and possessions that can quickly vanish. If such a loss does happen, the storm-struck victim may dream of an upside down tree, its roots reaching up to evanescent clouds. That terror of groundlessness is one of the darkest shadows of patriarchy. Science tries to compensate by trying to find facts. A darker, dangerous compensation is in the rejection of the feminine in body and nature where it is often dismissed as irrational, histrionic, flaky, touchy-feely—words that mock, reject, rape, personally and globally.

Nietzsche's paradox is a well-known truth to anyone who has been forced to travel the brutal and beautiful terrain of his or her own body when it is wandering in seemingly unexplained symptoms. In that wilderness, drums and active imagination provide the soul-map. Courage, patience, trust cut through the jungle. Every step affirms the paradox: the ascension to spirit demands the descent into ground. Ground in yoga is the *muladhara,* the root chakra in which one takes root in our own humanity through which we experience our own divinity.

Judith Harris's chapter titles announce her interest in bringing that paradox into experience in psyche and body: 1) Creation, 2) Body as Container, 6) Muladhara, Elephants and the Kabbala, 7) The Fire of Kundalini. As she articulates the vibration of her own experience, she affirms the essential role of body in bringing the energy inherent in symbols into life. Far from diminishing Jung's understanding of dreamwork, this book validates his understanding of the image as connector between soma and psyche and enhances his "knowing" of the totality of heart and head. *Jung and Yoga* is a genuine contribution to twenty-first century medicine.

Marion Woodman

Preface

For many years I sought a form of bodywork that I could incorporate into my daily life. Finally, in the late 1980s, I found myself living down the street from Esther Myers' Yoga Studio in Toronto. Yoga appealed to me as a possible path for bringing spirit into body in a balanced, conscious way. And so, my initiation into bodywork began.

Suddenly, I was faced with all my fears and inferiorities. Just to remain present for ninety minutes challenged me to the core of my being. Most of the time I would stay at the back of the class, unable to do much of what was being asked. After just a few months, with enormous help and guidance from my teacher, Esther Myers, I began to feel what it was like to be *in* my body for the first time. Whenever a loving hand was placed on my back, my body responded with deep gratitude. With the aid of the breath, the everlasting breath that transforms the body with consciousness, my spine slowly began to relax its locked rigidity.

A few years later, I went to Zurich to train as an analyst and simultaneously began to teach yoga to a small group of friends in my living room. Slowly the group grew, and it was these sacred Monday evenings that became the wellspring of my current practice and this book.

As I began to see analysands, I knew immediately and deeply that my analytic practice had to be grounded in the awareness of body. It is the conscious containing of both psyche and body that allows a dropping down to center, to that place of stillness within that will ultimately bring renewal.

Many of us have endured a life not-yet-lived. In this mysterious place between the opposites, we may finally find our own life. There, previously hidden energy brings psyche and body together, uniting them in the sacred union that gives birth to new consciousness, and the gift of a life fully lived.

Sources of Illustrations

See Bibliography for Publication details
CW refers to *The Collected Works of C.G. Jung*

1. *Psychology and Alchemy*, CW 12, fig. 163.
2. *Psychology and Alchemy*, CW 12, fig. 71.
3. M.V. Seton-Williams, *Egyptian Legends and Stories*, p. 63.
4. Analysand's drawing.
5. C.G. Jung, *Nietzsche's* Zarathustra, p. 1412.
6. *Psychology and Alchemy*, CW 12, fig. 78.
7. Mary Stewart, *Yoga*, p. 16.
8. Marie-Louise von Franz, *Number and Time*, p. 130.
9. *Mysterium Coniunctionis*, CW 14, p. 195.
10. Friedhelm Hardy, *The Religious Culture of India*, p. 25.
11. Friedhelm Hardy, *The Religious Culture of India*, p. 27.
12. Eric Franklin, *Dynamic Alignment Through Imagery*, p. 188.
13. Irene Dowd, *Taking Root to Fly*, p. 15.
14. Jill Purce, *The Mystic Spiral,* plate 45.
15. Vanda Scaravelli, *Awakening the Spine*, p. 12.
16. Vanda Scaravelli, *Awakening the Spine*, p. 13.
17. C.G. Jung, *The Psychology of Kundalini Yoga*, picture 2.
18. Heinrich Zimmer, *Myths and Symbols in Indian Art and Civilization*, pl. 26.
19. Roger Cook, *The Tree of Life*, p. 19
20. Allen Afterman, *Kabbala and Consciousness*, p. 93.
21. C.G. Jung, *The Visions Seminars*, vol. 1, plate 21.
22. *The Archetypes and the Collective Unconscious*, CW 9i, fig. 17.
23. C.G. Jung, *The Visions Seminars*, vol. 1, plate 12.
24. *Psychology and Alchemy,* CW 12, fig. 131.
25. Judith Anodea, *Wheels of Life*, p. 37.
26. Jill Purce, *The Mystic Spiral*, plate 11.
27. Judith Anodea, *Wheels of Life*, p. 39.
28. Jill Purce, *The Mystic Spiral,* plate 10.
29. David Gordon White, *The Alchemical Body*, p. 45.
30. *The Archetypes and the Collective Unconscious*, CW 9i, fig. 4.

1

Creation

In the beginning God created the heaven and the earth. And the earth
was without form and void; and darkness was on the face of the deep.
And a wind from God moved over the surface of the waters. And God
said, Let there be light; and there was light. And God saw the light,
that it was good: and God divided the light from the darkness. And
God called the light Day, and the darkness he called Night. And there
was evening and there was morning, one day.
—Genesis 1:1-5 (Jerusalem Bible).

Creation has begun. For centuries we have posed the questions: Did
anything exist before the beginnings of creation? Did God create the
heaven and the earth from nothing, from absolutely nothing? Apart
from God, did no other beings or life of any kind exist before the
heaven and the earth were created?

I have long pondered these questions. Avivah Gottlieb Zornberg
reminds us that Rashi (1040-1105), the foremost Judaic commentator
on the Torah (the five books of Moses, explains that the opening sentence of Genesis in fact tells us nothing about how the world actually
began.[1] Rashi comments that heaven and earth were not actually created first, nor were they created out of nothing, as many of us have
been taught and have always believed. Water simply appears in the
second verse. No account is actually given of water being created. We
can assume, therefore, that the waters have always been in existence.
This primal ocean existed long before what we call time began.

The second verse of Genesis tells us that a wind from God moved
over the surface of the waters. In other words, the divine spirit has
been in existence since eternity. As Jung explains:

The *anima mundi*, the demiurge or divine spirit that incubated the chaotic

---

[1] *Genesis: The Beginning of Desire*, pp. 3ff.

waters of the beginning, remained in matter in a potential state, and the initial chaotic condition persisted with it.[2]

This profound statement of Jung's speaks of the original human in a prenatal state, still identical with the unconscious. The first task that must be faced at the beginning of a personal analysis is the discovery of the *prima materia*, the original source in alchemy. This initial state remains hidden until, through the work of bringing unconscious material to consciousness, it reveals itself in its own time. Our work is to bring order and meaning to the chaos. The alchemists started with the *prima materia*, the dark, chaotic world which contains infinite possibilities and potentialities for creation. A Midrashic legend[3] helps us understand how the *prima materia* is created.[4]

The legend tells us that the light created out of the darkness on the first day of creation was an awesome primordial light seven times brighter than the light of the sun, which itself was not created until the fourth day. It is said that this primordial light shone uninterrupted over the whole seven days of creation and did not actually set until the end of the seventh day, until the conclusion of the first Sabbath, just before the cycle of the new week was to begin. This first darkness, however, was a great and terrible darkness.

The first man, Adam, was created on the sixth day, six being the first number that represents the sum of its divisions (1 + 2 + 3). It signifies a completeness; at the close of the sixth day creation was completed. The Midrash specifies that man was created on Friday afternoon, the afternoon of the sixth day. This is a very important time in Judaism for it is the afternoon before the eve of the Sabbath, the seventh day. It is said that on that same day, the same sixth day, Adam and Eve sinned by eating from the tree of knowledge. They were banished from the Garden of Eden on the sixth day, but, as the Sab-

---

[2] "The Terry Lectures," *Psychology and Religion*, CW 11, par. 160. (CW refers throughout to *The Collected Works of C.G. Jung*)

[3] A Midrash is a type of Judaic Biblical interpretation in which the text is explained differently from its literal meaning by bringing symbolic amplification to the original Biblical passage.

[4] Lawrence Kushner, *The River of Light*, p. 95.

bath was approaching, the great darkness did not descend on them until the close of the Sabbath, more than one day later. One might say they had been granted this extra day by the grace of God.

An extra soul comes down from heaven for the duration of the Sabbath every week and with it extra holiness is bestowed on us. This divine energy can be thought of as compensation for the sin which Adam and Eve had committed in the Garden. Therefore, they received this additional soul when they were granted the extra day in Paradise. The knowledge that they were endowed with this special day of holiness before being cast out into the darkness made this day even more special. However, with the birth of consciousness paradise was coming to an end, as it must for us all.

The everlasting light that had been shining consistently for seven days had been extinguished. And now, in the absence of light, Adam became aware that there was light. This shows us the fundamental paradoxical duality that brings forth consciousness. Adam had been plunged into darkness. Suffering must also accompany states of ecstasy, otherwise we would never understand what ecstasy is, just as Adam knew light only when there was light no longer. In consciousness, his suffering began. Alone in the newness of the night he lamented: "Woe to me. For now that I have defiled the world, this darkness is come upon it forever. Creation will revert to primordial chaos. Heaven has condemned me to death."[5]

In the midst of intense suffering we often feel that no light will ever come. We must realize that this depth of anguish was necessary for Adam at that time, so that with the birth of the new dawn (it is actually the first real dawn as there had not yet been darkness on the earth), the task of ordering the universe could begin. This legend, as retold in the Talmud (the most important work of the oral Torah) tells us the story of the creation and of the uncovering of the *prima materia*, the basis of all life.

What has actually occurred is that with the suffering that must accompany the birth of consciousness, Adam has been thrown back to

---

[5] Ibid., p. 96.

his chaotic beginnings where he enters the whole process again, this time on a different level, this time consciously. This is what is meant by the rediscovery of the *prima materia*.

After the *prima materia* has been found, the opposites must be separated out of the chaos in order that they may later be reunited in a new way. It is the breaking apart into opposites on which emergence into reality depends. The main task of the work is the reconciliation of the opposites leading to union with the divine principle. In the divine, all opposites are reunited.

> There is no consciousness without the discrimination of opposites. This is the paternal principle, the Logos, which eternally struggles to extricate itself from the primal warmth and primal darkness of the maternal womb; in a word, from unconsciousness. Divine curiosity yearns to be born and does not shrink from conflict, suffering, or sin. . . . Nothing can exist without its opposite; the two were one in the beginning and will be one again in the end. Consciousness can only exist through continual recognition of the unconscious, just as everything that lives must pass through many deaths.[6]

Edward Edinger explains consciousness beautifully by reminding us of the etymology:

> *Conscious* derives from *con* or *cum*, meaning "with" or "together," and *scire*, "to know," or "to see." It has the same derivation as *conscience*. Thus the root meaning of both consciousness and conscience is "knowing with" or "seeing with" an "other." In contrast, the word science, which also derives from *scire*, means simple knowing, i.e., knowing without "withness." So etymology indicates that the phenomena of consciousness and conscience are somehow related and that the experience of consciousness is made up of two factors—"knowing" and "withness." In other words, consciousness is the experience of *knowing together with an other*, that is, in a setting of twoness.[7]

Consciousness begins with the first sentence of Genesis: "In the

---

[6] "Psychological Aspects of the Mother Archetype," *The Archetypes and the Collective Unconscious*, CW 9i, par. 178.
[7] *The Creation of Consciousness: Jung's Myth for Modern Man,* p. 36.

beginning God created the heaven and the earth."

There are literally thousands of myths from all around the world that attempt to explain creation, the birth of the conscious world. The first poets, Vedic, Egyptian, Babylonian and Chinese, all pondered the mysteries of creation. Its myths refer to the most basic problems of human life, for they are concerned with the ultimate meaning of not only human existence, but that of the whole cosmos.[8]

A Chinese creation myth gives us a wonderful explanation of the original division of heaven and earth:

In the beginning there was a huge egg containing chaos, a mixture of yin-yang, female-male, cold-hot, dark-light and wet-dry. Within this egg was a giant called Phan-Ku who had not yet been anything but who now broke out of the egg, and it was he who separated the chaos into the many opposites including earth and sky. Each day thereafter, for the next 18,000 years, Phan Ku grew ten feet between the sky, which was raised ten feet, and the earth, which grew down ten feet. That is why heaven and earth, so it is said, are now separated by thirty thousand miles.[9]

When the opposites are thrown apart, space is created between them for consciousness to be born. When one lives in the chaotic state of undifferentiated opposites, a state of *participation mystique,* subject cannot be distinguished from object. This is the ideal paradisal state of the mother-infant relationship. Marie-Louise von Franz tells us that after the cosmic egg has been created it is generally divided into two parts, and that this same motif of separation of the preconscious unit appears frequently in connection with the separation of the first parents.[10] In many myths Father Heaven and Mother Earth exist in an embrace, forming an hermaphroditic being in constant cohabitation. In this state nothing can be born into existence, because Father Heaven is lying so closely with Mother Earth that there is no room for

---

[8] Marie-Louise von Franz, *Creation Myths*, p. 1.

[9] David Adams Leeming and Margaret Adams Leeming, *A Dictionary of Creation Myths*, p. 49.

[10] *Creation Myths*, p. 233.

anything to grow between them. There is no space whatsoever. Creation can only take place in the space formed by their separation. In other words, when one becomes conscious one is able to remain in the space between the opposites, able to contain and endure the tension between them. This is one of the major tasks of analysis, to separate subject from object and live no longer in infantile *participation mystique* with the surrounding world. As differentiation between subject and object occurs, the creation of the ego, of who I am, begins.

This initial state in analysis may be likened to the alchemical *prima materia*, an imperfect and dissociated state which must be worked on. In order to "work on" the *prima materia*, certain very important steps must be taken. The alchemists believed that transformation could not take place until the *prima materia* had been rediscovered. This means, analytically speaking, that we must go back and rediscover our original, uncontaminated state in order for a real transformation to occur. This cannot take place simply at the ego level, for there it will remain too superficial. Something else has to happen.

The *prima materia* signifies a multitude of things. In fact, paradoxically, it means everything, the beginning as well as the end of the work. What is most important, however, is that the *prima materia* is called *radix ipsius* (root of itself). As the *prima materia* is able to root within itself, it remains completely autonomous and dependent on nothing.[11] This is what allows it to be ever-present, in every way. We can think of it as the water that was present before God created heaven and earth. As the *prima materia* can root itself without any external forces acting upon it, we may also liken it to the earth. Indeed, Jung often refers to the *prima materia* as the earth (Figure 1) and calls it "the mother of the elements and of all created things."[12]

Jung speaks in this same paragraph of the *prima materia* as being something which is "uncreated." In other words, we go back to the idea that it need only be discovered in order for the process to begin—it has always existed and therefore does not need to be created.

---

[11] "The Prima Materia," *Psychology and Alchemy*, CW 12, par. 429.
[12] Ibid. par. 430.

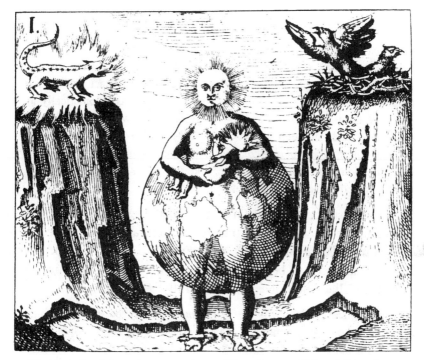

Figure 1. Earth as *prima materia*, suckling the son of the philosophers.

One could say that it is waiting to be found. This task of rediscovering the *prima materia* may be the most difficult task in the beginning of analysis. It may take years until vital contact is made.

Prima materia is the earth and earth is the basic substance of the human body. This tells us that the *prima materia* is, among other things, the human body.[13] Humankind is ashes and to ashes shall we return, as we read in Genesis where God gives his commandments after Adam and Eve had eaten of the tree of knowledge. God says:

> In the sweat of thy face shalt thou eat bread, till thou return to the ground; for out of it wast thou taken: for dust thou art, and to dust shalt thou return.[14]

---

[13] *Aurora Consurgens*, p. 343.
[14] Gen. 3:19. (Biblical references throughout are to the Jerusalem Bible)

Adam, in fact, is likened by Jung to the *prima materia:*

We must now turn to the question of why it was that Adam should have been selected as a symbol for the prima materia or transformative substance. This was probably due, in the first place, to the fact that he was made out of clay, the "ubiquitous" *materia vilis* that was axiomatically regarded as the prima materia and for that very reason was so tantalizingly difficult to find, although it was "before all eyes." It was a piece of the original chaos, of the *massa confusa,* not yet differentiated but capable of differentiation; something, therefore, like shapeless, embryonic tissue. Everything could be made out of it.[15]

In my experience, without this return to the original substance, to the earth and to the body, real transformation cannot take place. The body acts as the container of transformation. We must go back to our beginnings in order to be reborn. Our origins stretch back into eternity. Mircea Eliade describes this beautifully:

This alchemical reduction to the *prima materia* may be interpreted in a great variety of ways: notably it may be equated with a regression to the pre-natal state, a *regressus ad uterum* . . . According to Paracelsus, "he who would enter the Kingdom of God must first enter with his body into his mother and there die." The whole world, according to the same writer, must "enter into its mother," which is the *prima materia,* the *massa confusa,* the *abyssus,* in order to achieve eternity. . . . In the verses published as an appendix to the *Opus Mago-Cabbalisticum et Theosophicum* (1735) by Georg von Welling, we may read: "For I cannot otherwise reach the Kingdom of Heaven unless I am born a second time. Therefore I desire to return to the mother's womb, that I may be regenerated, and this I will do right soon." . . . The "mother" symbolizes, in these different contexts, nature in her primordial state, the *prima materia* of the alchemists, and the "return to the mother" translates a spiritual experience corresponding to any other "projection" outside Time—in other words, to the reintegration of a primal situation. The dissolution to the *prima materia* is also symbolized by a sexual union which is completed by disappearance into the uterus . . . the return to the seminal stage of existence.[16]

---

[15] "Adam and Eve," *Mysterium Coniunctionis,* CW 14, par. 552.
[16] Mircea Eliade, *The Forge and the Crucible,* p. 154ff.

Unfortunately, the body is often neglected in analysis. In 1946, Jung wrote a landmark paper that forms the bridge to his late works entitled "On The Nature Of The Psyche," in which he says that most probably psyche and body are two different aspects of one and the same thing.[17] Jung knew that they were essentially connected through reciprocal action, although the actual nature of this relationship was still completely outside his own experience. Since Jung died in 1961 it is becoming clearer how the interrelationship of the psyche and the body might actually take place. We must not forget, however, that Jung had already discovered a definite relationship between the two opposite ends of the spectrum, namely, the infrared, instinctual pole, and the ultraviolet, archetypal pole of the spectrum. Jung knew that these two aspects clearly belonged together but he also realized that this was as far as he himself could progress at that time and that he had to leave the research to those who would follow him. It is interesting that in Jung's Nietzsche seminars Barbara Hannah remarked: "You can be anything but you must stay in your body."[18]

Today, in the Jungian world, it is generally acknowledged that there is a body-psyche connection. Unfortunately, however, it is often assumed that if the psyche can be strengthened, it will simply carry the body along with it. In other words, it is thought that the psychic energy will penetrate the cells of the body, allowing transformation to take place in both realms at the same time. This implies, of course, that the body is secondary in importance to the psyche, as it would then just be "following along," so to speak. I consider this assumption to be false, as over and over again we can see that the body does not simply follow the progress of the psyche. It often has a "mind" of its own and needs to be treated accordingly. In my experience, the simultaneous transformation of the body and the psyche is only possible if both sides are worked on at the same time. In the East mind and body were never treated as separate entities. If one accepts Jung's theory of the opposites as a cosmic reality, then it would not be possible

---

[17] *The Structure and Dynamics of the Psyche*, CW 8, pars. 343ff.
[18] *Nietzsche's* Zarathustra: *Notes of the Seminar Given in 1934-1939*, p. 65.

to consider only one side to the exclusion of the other. It would be ludicrous to assume that the opposite would simply follow along in agreement. Both must therefore have an equal place in analysis.

The first time Jung mentions the word "archetype" in his writings is in the essay "Instinct and the Unconscious," written in 1919. Jung never doubted that instinct and archetype belong together. He describes archetypes and instincts as the most polar opposites imaginable, as can easily be seen when one compares a person who is ruled by instinctual drives with one who is seized by the spirit.

INSTINCTS	ARCHETYPES
infrared ———————————————————— ultraviolet	
(**Physiological:** body symptoms, instinctual perceptions, etc.)	(**Psychological:** spirit, dreams, conceptions, images, fantasies, etc.)

As opposites are always extreme qualities with a close bond between them, no position can actually be established, or even thought of, without its corresponding negation. As with any pairs of opposites, one can become possessed if too much energy is manifesting at one pole. For example, a person consumed by instinct might be controlled by obsessive sexuality or by food cravings, whereas to be possessed by the other pole, the pole of the archetypal or the spiritual, would mean being driven by, say, ideology. In either case, there is no freedom whatsoever.

Jung speaks of a place where the opposite poles of spirit and matter both meet and don't meet. This is the place that we would term today the "subtle body," the intermediate place between spirit and body, between the heavenly and earthly realms. Paracelsus, the Renaissance philosopher, stated that there exists another half of man, and that he does not consist of flesh and blood alone, but also of a body that cannot be discerned by human eyesight. It is in this place that body and spirit are united as one. It is said in ancient yogic teachings that this invisible subtle body is connected to our physical body by a slender silken cord. One might also say that the place of connection between the physical body and the subtle body is the soul. Jacob Boehme, a

German mystic and alchemist who died at the beginning of the seventeenth century and whose ideas exerted a significant influence on Jung, particularly in regard to the symbolism of the mandala, writes:

> The soul has its origins not only from the body, though it taketh its rise in the body, and has its first beginnings in the body; yet it hath also its source from without, by and from the air; and so the Holy Ghost ruleth in it, in that manner as he replenisheth and filleth all things.[19]

It is here in the subtle body that the psyche and the body have a mutual influence. The body will exhibit symptoms until the psyche becomes strong enough to contain and carry the conflict.

Jung tells us that instincts and archetypes together form the collective unconscious, meaning that both are universal and regularly occurring phenomena which have essentially nothing to do with individuality. He says further that one cannot deal with instincts, per se, without considering the archetypes, because in the end they determine one another and have a reciprocal influence.

The first experience we have in this world is of the mother, the personal as well as the archetypal mother. We are attached to her body, first inside her womb and then we are born out of her body into the world. This physical and emotional contact with the mother's body remains crucial and influences us forever, whether or not she has been present to us with her body, whether or not we experience her body as positive or negative. The archetype of the mother is constellated at conception:

> "Mother" is an archetype and refers to the place of origin, to nature, to that which passively creates, hence to substance and matter, to materiality, the womb, the vegetative functions. It also means the unconscious, our natural and instinctive life, the physiological realm, the body in which we dwell or are contained; for the "mother" is also the matrix, the hollow form, the vessel that carries and nourishes, and it thus stands psychologically for the foundation of consciousness.[20]

---

[19] Quoted in David V. Tansley, *Subtle Body: Essence and Shadow*, p. 20.
[20] "The Practical Use of Dream-Analysis," *The Practice of Psychotherapy*, CW 16, par. 344.

In Jung's view the psyche consists of both the archetypal realm and the instinctual world of matter. He says:

> Since psyche and matter are contained in one and the same world, and moreover are in continuous contact with one another and ultimately rest on irrepresentable, transcendental factors, it is not only possible but fairly probable, even, that psyche and matter are two different aspects of one and the same thing. The synchronicity phenomena point, it seems to me, in this direction, for they show that the non-psychic can behave like the psychic, and vice versa, without there being any causal connection between them. Our present knowledge does not allow us to do much more than compare the relation of the psychic to the material world with two cones, whose apices, meeting in a point without extension—a real zero-point— touch and do not touch.[21]

To neglect the body is to neglect half of our world. It is to neglect from whence we come, the *prima materia*. It disregards our connection to earth, to matter, to the world of nature and to the feminine. To overlook the archetypal world is to dismiss the possibility of healing. Both aspects are needed for transformation. The psyche must include the entire spectrum, from instinct to archetype.

---

[21] "On the Nature of the Psyche," *The Structure and Dynamics of the Psyche,* CW 8, par. 418.

2
The Body As Container

Know the Self as lord of the chariot,
The body as the chariot itself,
The discriminating intellect as charioteer,
And the mind as reins.
—Katha Upanishad 3.3.

Occasionally we are lucky enough to find the *prima materia* at the beginning of analysis. The work of transformation can then begin immediately. Why this occurs in only some cases remains a mystery, but I suspect it may have something to do with the extent of suffering that the analysand brings at the outset. There seems, then, to be no choice but to dive, so to speak, into the unconscious. Of course, in these cases it must be carefully assessed whether or not the ego is strong enough to take this initial intensity, for sometimes the analysand must bear even more suffering as consciousness emerges.

Often, however, there is no choice. Fate has brought this virtually intolerable suffering as the impetus toward consciousness is constellated. It is important to remember, as M. Esther Harding notes, that there is an innate drive within us toward wholeness:

The task of becoming whole is one that cannot be ignored. . . . Thus certain persons find themselves obliged to undertake the task of individuation as a conscious willed enterprise, even though the quest promises no definite ending. Once it is undertaken, however, aid comes from an unexpected source, namely the unconscious itself. For symbols of wholeness begin to appear in dreams and phantasies and in other products of the unconscious, pointing the way that must be taken, even if this way leads towards an unknown goal. Thus the quest for wholeness shows itself to be in line with an archetypal trend inherent in the psychic structure of the human being. This trend is akin to an instinct and, like the instincts, is capable of showing the way to be taken by the developing organism.[22]

---

[22] *Psychic Energy: Its Source and Transformation*, pp. 339f.

This innate striving for wholeness brings us closer to who we actually are, the one we were created to become.

June came into analysis just after her twenty-first birthday. At the time she was in a very critical state, suffering from neurodermatitis, a condition which produces chronic severe inflammation of the skin. June was no longer recognizable as a young woman but looked instead like a withered, sick old lady. Her eyes were ringed by several swollen circles, making it scarcely possible to make eye contact with her. The disease covered her body from her head to just above her ankles. The skin on her neck had become so thick that she could barely move her head from side to side. She was completely exhausted from lack of sleep—the scratching was incessant. Her skin was so deeply cut and wounded that the smell of blood was evident from the moment she entered my room. She had come into analysis to investigate the possible psychosomatic component of the disease, as well as to get help in dealing with her acute distress.

June was desperate. She had tried various medical therapies for about half a year including spending several months in a skin clinic in Germany. She had used so much cortisone that it had begun to lose its effectiveness. Long-term use of cortisone actually causes the skin itself to become very thin, reducing even further its natural ability to serve as a semi-permeable filter between the inner and outer worlds. June had begun to dislike drug therapy, had become afraid of the long-term effects, and had therefore stopped using cortisone just a few weeks before our first meeting. The skin disease had worsened as she stopped taking the cortisone, but not considerably.

June had been told by her dermatologist that she would not get better unless she continued to take the cortisone in large amounts, internally as well as topically. From a wholly different perspective, however, I remembered that a symptom is a natural attempt on the part of the psyche toward healing, toward wholeness. I felt very strongly that the symptom manifesting in this unbearable skin disease was, paradoxically, a step toward healing. Disease is often the stimulus that can bring transformation. Hence Jung reminds us of "the fundamental principle that the symptomatology of an illness is at the same time a natural attempt at healing."[23]

It seemed likely to me that whatever was too painful for June to bring to consciousness was coming up instead in an indirect way, as a bodily symptom. The psychic structure was too weak to hold the conflict, whatever that was, so the conflict had entered her body. In fact, when an illness manifests itself in the body it is easier to deal with, though the symptoms can be torturous. When the illness is in the psyche, however, it is invisible and harder to treat. June's illness was now manifesting in the infrared side of the spectrum, the body side. In fact she was being forced to deal directly with the color red, manifesting in redness as well as the terrible bleeding of her skin. The instinctual realm was literally crying out to be heard, for the integration of instinct is essential to the process of individuation.

Cortisone is known to be an immune suppressant, thereby reducing the production of the natural "killer cells" in the body. We need these natural fighters to combat disease and it is known that serious medical problems can result from the long term ingesting of cortisone. I believed that the skin disease was the manifestation of something psychic trying to find expression in this bodily symptom, and since taking cortisone would only further suppress this ability as well as reduce June's ability to resist other illnesses, I decided to support her attempt, against medical advice, to find another way of healing. When I look back, I feel this was a big step in our deciding together to deal with what could possibly come up from the unconscious. First we had to deal with the skin disease becoming even worse, however, for the attempt at healing, at becoming conscious, was becoming ever more urgent.

We had only two hours together and then June went on holiday. Before she left, I asked her if she would like to take some clay with her. June promptly took a knife, sliced the clay in half on my table, and asked if she could have half of it, saying that she would leave the other half with me for when she came back. The skin is the organ of

---

[23] "The Structure of the Psyche," *The Structure and Dynamics of the Psyche*, CW 8, par. 312.

touch, actually the organ of feeling, as we feel things with our hands. It seemed June had received very little real feeling from her mother. Her mother came from a very high-class Chinese family where spontaneity, warmth and physical contact had been lacking. June had not been a wanted child. Her parents had married because of the pregnancy, and both sets of grandparents were ashamed of the marriage. June's birth had not been celebrated. As Marion Woodman tells us:

> A mother who cannot welcome her baby girl into the world leaves her daughter groundless. Similarly, the mother's mother and grandmother were probably without the deep roots that connect a woman's body to earth. Whatever the cause, her own instinctual life is unavailable.[24]

In fact, when June first became seriously ill, her mother had applied the cortisone cream to her body while wearing thick latex gloves. June said she wished she could have had the real touch from her mother, especially when she was so ill. I felt that working with the clay could be the beginnings of coming into contact with something of the earth, of the *prima materia*, of the Great Mother. Clay would be something she would be able to take in her own hands and mold herself.

What June actually needed was to create a new, transformed body for herself. In doing so, she would be able to bring the disconnected parts of herself together, and spirit and body would become one. I felt that working with clay could support such a transformation. In alchemy the goal of the work is the transformation of base metals into gold, which is considered to be the ultimate result of a long period of gestation in the bowels of the earth. The gold in the opus is the subtle body. The transformed body would therefore represent for June the connection to the eternal part of herself, thereby allowing the body itself to undergo profound change. As a matter of fact June's skin completely cleared after about eight months of analysis.

We find many situations similar to this young woman's, where the experience of the mother archetype has been primarily negative. The mother-child relationship at the beginning of life is absolutely vital to

---

[24] *The Ravaged Bridegroom: Masculinity in Women*, p. 74.

the future development of the child. D.W. Winnicott describes this as "primary maternal preoccupation." In other words, the mother must develop a conscious, but also a deeply unconscious, identification with her infant:

> The mother who develops this state that I have called "primary maternal preoccupation" provides a setting for the infant's constitution to begin to make itself evident, for the developmental tendencies to start to unfold, and for the infant to experience spontaneous movement and become the owner of the sensations that are appropriate to this early phase of life.[25]

We can see clearly from this statement how the failure to relate to the body can originate.

In using the clay I had given her, June would be working with the *prima materia;* she would be working with the place in time before we were born, before karma and the experience of life brings our fate to us. She would be going gently back to the place before time began, bringing profound healing to her deep wounding in the instinctual, body realm. Kneading clay is working on the body. We read in the Bible that the first man, Adam, was made out of the dust of the earth (Figure 2). Earth mixed with water produces clay. In a seventeenth-century alchemical text it is written: "When the water fell upon the earth, Adam was created."[26]

In fact, June would be working directly with her illness by using clay. In ancient times, the skin was equated with the soul. June would actually be working with her afflicted soul, as it was manifesting in her body, through the process of kneading and molding the clay.

June was reeling between the opposites of life and death. She shared an excerpt from her journal with me at that time:

> I CAN'T TAKE THIS ANYMORE!! I WANT ANOTHER SKIN. IT HAS BECOME SO THICK. THE ITCHING IS UNBEARABLE. WHY AM I BEING PUNISHED IN THIS WAY?? WHAT MUST I DO IN ORDER TO BE FREED FROM THIS HELLISH TORTURE?? WHY

---

[25] Winnicott, *Through Paediatrics to Psychoanalysis,* p. 303.
[26] *Theatr. chem.,* V, p. 109, quoted in *Mysterium Coniunctionis,* CW 14, par. 552.

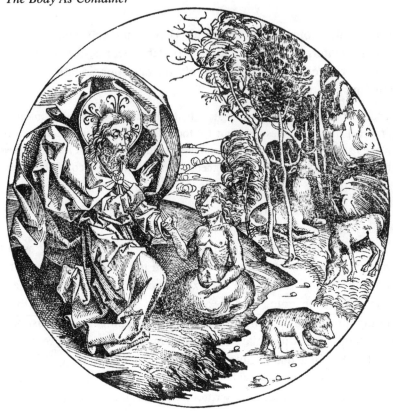

Figure 2. The creation of Adam from the clay of the *prima materia.*

DOESN'T ANYBODY HELP ME? I CAN'T BEAR IT. I WANT TO
SCRATCH ALL MY SKIN OFF. I CAN'T TAKE IT ANYMORE, I
CAN'T ENDURE IT ONE DAY LONGER.

June and I both knew that something huge had to happen to relieve
her suffering. Often we must go to the depths in order for things to
change. With all the scratching and bleeding, she was losing much of
her old skin. She was going to have to let go of an old attitude and
somehow begin to embrace something new. Analysis does not "cure"
people, per se. It is rather more accurate to speak of a readjustment of
attitude; in other words, a new way of looking at one's life slowly
emerges with time. June was literally going to have to shed her old
attitudes, her old skin, so to speak, in order for transformation to be

possible. She was going to have to make a huge decision, for if she were not willing to let go of some of her old attitudes toward her own life as well as toward the world around her, psychic or even physical death could result. Fortunately, there was a readiness in her, and our work began with a passionate intensity.

The fact that June was specifically afflicted with a skin disease was no coincidence. Skin is associated with the ideas of birth and rebirth. In the Egyptian system of hieroglyphs there is a sign comprising three skins knotted together, signifying "to be born"; it comes into the composition of words such as "to engender," "to bring up," and "to form." The amulet which the Egyptians used to present to new-born children comprised, like the hieroglyph, three animal pelts which were attached to a solar globe. The number of the skins here refers to the essentially threefold nature of the human being—body, soul and spirit—while the globe denotes one's incorporation into the All. The symbolism of the skin is borne out by the rite known as "the passage through the skin" which pharaohs and priests used to carry out in order to rejuvenate themselves.[27]

Another analysand, Susan, twenty-two years old, suddenly began having skin problems as the severe eating disorder of bulimia began to heal. In her case, however, the swelling, redness and itching disappeared fairly quickly as she had already been in analysis for two years when the skin symptoms appeared. During a bodywork session which took place at the time when the symptoms appeared she had a vision:

> I see a clear picture of three Egyptian women that suddenly changes into a most beautiful peaceful vision of a pottery room containing three clay ovens. These ovens are joined together at the top where they become one.

The image of the clay ovens was almost identical to the Egyptian hieroglyph. When Susan brought this image into the hour, I asked her if it was possible that she was growing a "new skin." In astonishment, she told me that her entire skin had been peeling off during the last forty-eight hours!

---

[27] J.E. Cirlot, *A Dictionary of Symbols*, pp. 298ff.

Susan had come into analysis in a very fragile state, with almost no ability to stand conflict. She was too "thin-skinned." Since that particular vision Susan has become visibly stronger. She is in fact growing a new skin, a new ability to deal with the world around her. Her delicate feminine soul shines through a skin that radiates life. Through this vision, which took place during a bodywork session, Susan is building a container where she can begin to hold intense conflict for the first time. The skin is the largest organ in the body and not only surrounds the entire body but also serves as a protection from the outside world. As Susan is now able to differentiate what she will let in from the outside world, her feelings of constantly being overwhelmed and unable to cope with life are lessening.

This vision also shows us the development of the feminine which had been constellated during the bodywork session. The first image that came to Susan was of Egyptian women. The fact that these women were Egyptian is particularly interesting. As an aside it should be noted that, as in this case, it very often happens that in visions or dreams, archetypal images come to us spontaneously, although there had been no previous conscious awareness of the image.

In most world mythologies the earth is considered feminine, as belonging to Mother Nature, and the sky, as spirit, is masculine. In Egypt, however, these concepts of masculine and feminine are reversed. Geb, the earth principle, is a male god and Nut is the sky goddess. In explaining this unusual phenomenon Marie-Louise von Franz tells us that in Egypt the concreteness of ideas is emphasized. All cultures, she tells us, hope for immortal life after death, but only in Egypt is the idea expressed through the preservation of the body in the quite concrete form of mummification.[28] The search for eternal life was also the quest of the early alchemists for something which could survive death. Psychologically, we would call this aspect the Self, that which is central and everlasting in us.

Susan grew up in a strong collective atmosphere where the body was regarded as something either to be gotten rid of, or to be put on

---

[28] *The Feminine in Fairy Tales*, p. 108.

display as ideal, not to be cherished as sacred. As Woodman so aptly puts it:

> Many people in our society are being driven to addictions because there is no collective container for their natural spiritual needs. Their natural propensity for transcendent experience, for ritual, for connection to some energy greater than their own, is being distorted into addictive behaviour.[29]

The vision of the pottery room containing three clay ovens harks back to the primordial man made out of clay which is capable of birthing a new, transformed body.

Peter dreamed a similar image after attending his regular yoga class. His mother had recently died and shortly thereafter he developed itchy, scaly red patches all over his legs. After the following dream the skin symptoms greatly lessened, although they have never completely disappeared.

> I am in a car with my mother and father and we have to get somewhere. I think it is to a synagogue. We stop the car and a couple of my friends get in and we continue on driving looking for this synagogue. I believe I am now driving the car. I am driving down many streets that are under repair until we finally come to an open square in a city that I don't recognise. At first I think it must be Jerusalem but then I see a big building with several domes on top, ornately decorated, like in India. Then I realize that I am in India.
>
> I still have not found the synagogue that I am looking for but now I realize that I had better get to my yoga class so as not to be late. I am now alone in the car and think that it is now time to get out of the car and get to my class.
>
> I find a small room in which the yoga class is taking place. My wife is standing at the front door waiting for me and beckoning me to come in. My teacher (my analyst) is in the inner part of the room. This room contains three brick ovens that resemble pizza ovens, strangely joined together at the top, and in each one a fire is going.

Up until this point, Peter had repressed his emotions, particularly his rage toward his dead mother who, on the one hand, had aban-

---

[29] *Addiction to Perfection: The Still Unravished Bride*, p. 29.

doned him through dying and, on the other hand, had left him free. Peter suffers from a very strong negative mother complex. As Peter's mother's behavior toward him had always alternated between invasion and rejection, relationship is particularly difficult for him. When he started coming to my yoga class a few years ago, Peter began to feel that yoga was helping to bring him closer to himself, to me as his analyst, and to God. In this dream one can see that positive mother has been constellated in the image of me as analyst being in the inner cave-room where the yoga class will take place. In the lysis (the end of the dream which tells us where the energy wants to go), it is clear here that a rebirth through the analytic container is possible. The image of the three pizza ovens coming together at the top again reminds us of the ancient Egyptian hieroglyph. Also, the number three signifies the resolution of the tension of the opposites. Maria Prophetissa tells us that three denotes the masculine, the fatherly and the spiritual.[30] Fire, the image of creation, denotes the masculine, as indicated by Jung:

> Fire is active, spiritual, emotional, close to consciousness, whereas water is passive, material, cool, and of the nature of the unconscious. Both are necessary to the alchemical process since this is concerned with the union of opposites.[31]

The energy in the unconscious is moving toward the masculine as contained within the feminine. The birth of the new feminine takes place through the bodywork, in this case through the practice of yoga.

Anne Maguire, analyst and physician, tells us that the archetype of fire as it appears in both ancient pictures and instinctive reactions comes to us in order to promote the healing of the skin of the afflicted. The archetype of fire manifests in the skin disease, bringing heat and pain in order to lead the afflicted person to a level of consciousness where the psychic difficulties that lie behind the disease can be recognized. As the skin is the mirror of the soul, so fire and emotion enter one's life. Without emotional life, there is neither light nor

---

[30] See "Introduction to the Religious and Psychological Problems of Alchemy," *Psychology and Alchemy*, CW 12, par. 31.
[31] "Paracelsus As A Spiritual Phenomenon," *Alchemical Studies*, CW 13, par. 187n.

life. Only through conflict can we begin to see the meaning of skin affliction. Emotion becomes our carrier of consciousness.[32]

June's illness had brought her life to a critical point. Fate had brought her to the place where she had to consciously make the decision whether she wanted to live or die. June was being tested in the fire of neurodermatitis. Anne Maguire compares the blisters that are symptomatic of this disease to tiny volcanoes which are on the point of breaking through the skin. She also tells us that the damage to the person with this illness is comparable to that of a volcano. When a volcano erupts, excess pressure and tension are discharged from the bowels of the earth. One can also speak of an increase in the inner psychic tension when an archetype is constellated in the unconscious. Jung describes an archetype as a core dynamic in the psyche that brings with it a huge quantity of energy.[33] The human skin serves as a safety valve as does the earth's crust, and it allows, through this dynamic, an eczematous discharge, comparable to that of a volcano. Maguire tells us that persons who are exhibiting such dermatological symptoms must look concurrently to a psychic factor, not as the cause, but rather as a connection. We are dealing here with what Jung would call synchronicity, a unique act of creation in time.

By the time June returned from her holidays, her skin had considerably worsened. She was hardly sleeping at all, literally wavering between life and death, unable to work or go to school. She could barely get to analysis. A few days before June returned she had this dream:

> I am a potter and a painter and I am exhibiting my clay and white plaster figures and paintings. In the figures as well as in the paintings there were images of my skin disease.

Although June had not used the clay I had given her, she had kept it with her all the time. With this initial dream, the *prima materia* had been constellated. A rebirth of the old consciousness that would lead into something new and alive was needed. Her unconscious had taken her back to the beginnings of time.

---

[32] *Hauterkrankungen als Botschaft der Seele* (The Fire and the Serpent), p. 268.
[33] "Definitions," *Psychological Types*, CW 6, pars. 747ff.

The alchemists believed that transformation could not begin to take place until the original state of *prima materia* had been reached. Here we can clearly see that the illness, the skin disease, is the stimulus that will bring profound change. June's body will be the carrier of this transformation.

This dream takes us back to Egypt around three thousand years before Christ, where the god Khnemu (often referred to as Khnum today) was worshipped as the "builder" of gods and men. He was often associated with Ptah, the great creator god. Together they worked to help create the universe. Ptah was concerned with constructing the heavens and the earth, while Khnemu was engaged in forming humans and animals. Ptah was often seen standing with an obelisk (a stone pillar having a square or rectangular cross-section and sides that taper toward a pyramidal top) at his back which not only acted as a stabilizing force but also symbolized the tree trunk in which the body of Osiris was hidden by Isis.[34] In being aligned with the earth, he was able to go through the cycle of death and rebirth as had Osiris before him.

Khnemu, on the other hand, created the first human beings on a potter's wheel, and it was said that he continued to "build up" their bodies and maintain their life.[35] Khnemu is shown in Figure 3 making two children at the same time: he is bringing the human being to consciousness. By using clay to form man, he was combining the primeval elements of earth and water. June had dreamt that her task was to create a new body, so to speak, by using the elements of earth and water in the form of clay.

Clay becomes three-dimensional when it becomes a body. Paradoxically, the white plaster figures contain all the possibilities of the creation of a new body, while also representing an old, worn-out body that can no longer live and must therefore be discarded in order for renewal to take place.

The fact that these plaster figures appear in white is very significant.

---

[34] E.A. Wallis Budge, *The Gods of the Egyptians*, vol. 1, pp. 501ff.
[35] Ibid, vol. 2, p. 50.

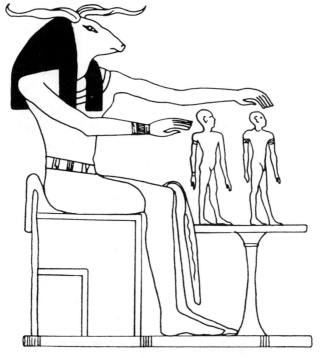

Figure 3. Khnemu at his potter's wheel.

White is the color of rebirth. At a wedding white symbolizes the death of the old life and birth into a new one. In ancient Greece, white clay was used by the priestesses of Artemis Alpheia at Letrini and Ortygia to daub their faces in honor of the White Goddess.[36] In death, white represents birth into the afterlife. White can also mean the absence of feeling, leading to a soul-death. Feeling had been almost completely absent in June's family; there had been no place at all for the development of the feminine, for Eros as relationship.

Another aspect of white is explained by Jung:

That it turns to white means that it becomes light. What has been unconscious life now becomes light, or understanding, consciousness. She

---

[36] See Robert Graves, *Greek Myths*, pp. 85ff.

should become conscious in an entirely new way, she should be conscious of life, as well as of things, in complete distinctness. A white light is supposed to be the brightest light, and that gives the power of discrimination, one can distinguish best then.[37]

Relatedness does not mean a merging, but rather a separateness allowing genuine experience of the other. The white figures in June's initial dream foreshadow a new consciousness. The situation had become urgent. The time had come for June to work with and integrate her body consciously, in analysis, as these clay and plaster figures indicated. Whitening, or *albedo* in alchemy, is the first stage of becoming aware of the autonomy of the objective psyche. It is the first stage of becoming conscious. A new attitude was decidedly called for. In truth, she had no choice.

Susan, the analysand with bulimia mentioned earlier, had an initial dream that presented quite a different image of the *prima materia*:

> I picked something up out of the water—it was an amoeba-like creature, long with a head but no arms or legs. The head was the head of my husband but something had happened to it and it was not very well.

Here we can see that the dreamer picks a content out of the unconscious that has not yet formed as a structure. Susan's relationship to her own body had been severely distorted. This left her with no place for her spiritual nature to grow in a healthy way, lovingly contained and held by the arms of the Great Mother. Her own father has suffered from severe depression for years. Susan's analytical work has consisted primarily of finding a structure that truly belongs to her, which allows her movement and freedom, in contrast to these initial images of the amoeba-like creature with no arms or legs. As Susan is finding her relationship to her long-lost body and the spirits within her, the bulimia has practically ceased.

---

[37] *The Visions Seminars*, p. 341.

3
"I Want To Be a Bird"

One bird tied up is better than one hundred in the air.
—Talmud, Ecclesiastes Rabbah 4:9.

When I met June for the first time she told me that all she had ever wanted in life was to be a bird. This seemed paradoxical to me, as birds often represent a desire to be out of life; they live high up where humans cannot go, and can also signify death when they appear in a dream.[38] I became aware in those first moments that this statement was actually the key to her illness. June had no desire to be part of the real world. She brought drawings with her to the first analytic hour that she had made the previous summer which clearly depicted her intense wish to die. These drawings had no color; they were only black, white and gray. At that time she was in bed most of the day, getting up occasionally to see a friend or to come to analysis. June had withdrawn from her studies and was also unable to go to work. Previously, she had been extremely successful and ambitious in all of her activities, both academically and in her personal life. Now she was reduced to doing almost nothing.

This is a common pattern also found in Chronic Fatigue Syndrome and Candida[39] as well as in related immune disorders. The desire and high expectations of achievement and success can flip the other way[40] and literally become inertia. June's desire to be a bird had left her

---

[38] See Marie-Louise von Franz, *On Dreams and Death*, p. 70.

[39] These two disorders are often related. Candida is a condition found in both men and women where there is an overgrowth of yeast in the body that can lead to chronic fatigue, allergies and emotional problems, as well as many other related symptoms that may or may not be incapacitating to the sufferer.

[40] This phenomenon is called *enantiodromia*, which means that everything will eventually turn into its opposite. It occurs mainly when there has been a tendency for a one-sided attitude to dominate consciousness.

helpless and incapacitated as a woman living in the world. As Marion Woodman explains, June had lost the precious connection to the earth, and therefore to her body, while flitting about in her fantasy world:

> The eagle represents the spiritual ascendancy of consciousness in its positive aspect; in its negative aspect, that ascendancy overreaches itself and becomes domination over and against that which belongs to the earth.[41]

Birds offer a clear distinction to snakes, for example. Snakes need no arms or legs because their spines are so flexible that their ribs are able to pull their bodies along the ground; for their motion they depend on the friction between the ground and the scales on the underside of their body. In taking to the air, birds exchanged a flexible spine for a rigid one. Birds have light, hard and relatively hollow bones and extremely strong forearms, while their legs are almost completely ignored except as accessories.[42] We humans need our legs and feet to support us on the ground. It is the flexibility of the spine that allows us freedom and a feeling of being secure on the earth. The spine supports us to stand erect in the world—the backbone of our existence. Without it, we would crumble.

June's birdlike body also manifested in tremendous fear and anxiety. Her skin had become like the spine of a bird, thick and rigid, as if she were in a condition near death. The thickening of the skin had predominated in the neck and throat area as the connection from her head to her body was almost nonexistent.

At the beginning of the analysis June had immediately asked to do bodywork. I knew then that the intensity of bodywork would be too much for her, in fact dangerous. I felt that it was too early to touch her since her illness was manifesting in the skin, the organ of touch. Touching her before real trust could be built between us, and before we had a chance to see what this skin disease might mean, could make things even worse, both with regard to the conscious problem of the skin disease itself and also with regard to bringing material up from the unconscious too soon. The psyche has its own timing. I decided,

---

[41] Marion Woodman and Elinor Dickson, *Dancing in the Flames*, p. 56.
[42] See Mabel Todd, *The Thinking Body*, p. 13.

therefore, to start the bodywork in a rather unusual way.

June and I actually began the bodywork sessions while she was sitting in her chair. I suggested the chair because I felt the floor or even a couch could have brought up the material from the unconscious too quickly, thus possibly making the skin disease even worse, which we could not risk. The disease was so acute at this point that June was at times delirious from lack of sleep. She was so exhausted in these early weeks of analysis and her anxiety level was so high, that she sometimes arrived for her hour, sat down in the chair, and said: "Oh good, I'm here now." Then she would lean back and close her eyes for some time before words could begin to speak her truth. I felt this to be a very positive sign for a strong healing potential as she was beginning to connect to a deep, archaic, preverbal state during this time. We would consciously prolong these states from time to time and I would simply follow her breathing, the inhalation and the exhalation, as she relaxed back into the chair.

Occasionally June would even fall asleep and when she awoke fifteen or so minutes later, she would seem refreshed and revitalized, with a little more energy than before. It was clear to me that she was back in a very early place at these times, back in the womb before her birth, or perhaps even back to a time that predated her conception. Nonetheless, June remained contained within the chair. There is always a certain danger with these sorts of people, those who have little or no footing on the ground, of falling into the unconscious. Jung describes this danger clearly in his Nietzsche seminars:

> Then Zarathustra simply carries a corpse and has no relation to life; he is without physical feet, a *pied à terre*, and therefore he loses reality. As a man, he loses touch with earth, he is always threatened with insanity.[43]

Sitting in a chair rather than on the floor in a traditional yoga posture can also have a grounding effect in cases where in the beginning stages there is almost no ground. This notion can seem confusing as one might think that sitting on the ground would provide the neces-

---

[43] *Nietzsche's* Zarathustra, p. 169.

sary grounding. But sitting on the ground can sometimes bring about fast and deep regression before one is ready.

Simply sitting and breathing in a chair with one's feet and heels firmly on the ground proved extremely valuable in June's situation. I began slowly by simply following her breathing, as she inhaled and exhaled. As with the yogic method of breathing, *pranayama*, I was able to bring the rhythm into a slow and quiet breath. Besides the natural consequence of relieving anxiety, the breathing is then able to go deeper and thereby penetrate more efficiently at the cellular level in the body. Transformation can take place at the cellular level through the fullest experience of the archetypal realm. It is ultimately the breath, the inhalation and exhalation, that unites microcosm to macrocosm. Through the breath we are joined to the Absolute, and it is for this reason in particular that control of the breath plays such a vital role in yoga practice.

The goal of this respiration, according to Taoist sources, is to imitate the respiration of the fetus in the maternal womb. "By returning to the base, by going back to the origin, one drives away old age, one returns to the state of the fetus."[44]

This is actually a special kind of breathing that I use only for such purposes, that is, to bring the analysand back into the womb in order that he or she may experience the mother archetype in a totally new way. Thus the *prima materia* is constellated. Ge Hong's *Baopuzi*, a Chinese alchemical text of the fourth century, speaks of longevity and immortality, and of embryo respiration as being the most significant way to achieve that end.[45] This type of rhythmic breathing was part of the discipline of the alchemist.

Another aspect of the discipline of the alchemist was the regulation of the transformative fire; in different stages of the process the fire must be different and the stages must be followed very carefully. The yogin strives to attain a state of "inner heat," which is then translated

---

[44] From the preface to the *T'ai-si K'ou Chueeh* ("Oral Formulas for Embryonic Respiration"), quoted in Mircea Eliade, *Yoga: Immortality and Freedom,* p. 67.

[45] Livia Kohn, *Taoist Meditation and Longevity Techniques,* p. 287.

to mean a mastery over the fire within. This is one of the most typical techniques employed in tantric yoga to achieve a magical production of heat, which in turn is assumed to transform the mortal body into an eternal spirit-body, that is, into subtle body. This "inner heat," or "mystical heat," is creative; one Indian myth even states that the world was created by the god Prajapati heating himself to an extreme degree by a kind of magical sweating. The tradition of the sweat lodge also serves the purpose of trying to attain this condition of excess heat. In ancient times this heat was obtained either by meditating close to a fire or by holding the breath. Various breathing practices, which included "embryonic respiration" as well as retention of the breath in order to produce intense heat, were held in high esteem as integral to mystical techniques.[46] Psychologically, heating the body can be understood as an intensification of consciousness.

Embryonic respiration is in fact a departure from the collective way of breathing; it is disciplined and rhythmic, rather than unconscious and irregular as our "natural" breathing tends to be:

> In the practice of embryo respiration, one does not use the nose or the mouth. Instead one breathes in the manner of an embryo inside the womb; who realizes this has truly attained the Tao.[47]

Interestingly, Taoists often place their dead before burial in the embryonic position with the hope of rebirth.

If this breathing practice can be attained, one begins to feel contained within the womb of the positive mother. Trust in life begins in such a loving container. June was becoming connected to the universal love of the mother through breathing with me. As Jung says:

> I understand the unconscious rather as an *impersonal* psyche common to all men, even though it expresses itself through a personal consciousness. When anyone breathes, his breathing is not to be interpreted personally.[48]

---

[46] Mircea Eliade, *Shamanism*, pp. 412ff.
[47] Ute Engelhardt, *Qi for Life: Longevity in the Tang*, quoted in Livia Kohn, *Taoist Meditation and Longevity Techniques,* p. 287.
[48] "The Psychological Aspects of the Kore," *The Archetypes and the Collective Unconscious*, CW 9i, par. 314.

And so the bodywork began.

Yoga is one of six systems of Indian philosophy. In Sanskrit, the word *yoga* means "to bind, join, attach, and yoke, to direct and concentrate one's attention on, to use and apply."[49] It is most often understood as the union of the individual with the transcendental self, with what Jung terms the Self. Here we come to a difficult place in understanding. Today, in this new millennium, many people in the Western world are searching for *nirvana*, the extinction of suffering, a way out of life. Yoga is usually thought of as a vehicle for transcending human experience, for attaining the absolute and leaving the material world behind. This is not practical for most Western minds. I am dealing here rather with a system of yoga conceived initially by Patanjali in the second century.

Patanjali, along with the Tantrists who succeeded him, was in fact searching for freedom, but not freedom from the reality of this world as we know it. We must remember that what is fundamental is experience. Experience comes naturally from knowing life in a concrete way, not just from following a spiritual path that excludes life itself. Liberation is thought of as liberation from ignorance; aspiration toward states of consciousness is foremost. Knowledge is liberation. Tantric yoga, in particular, places a high value on experience, bodily, practical and concrete, experience which, in combination with knowledge, will liberate us.

We come here to a very interesting point. Mircea Eliade points out that experience is essential to freedom, but in order to experience one must have a body.[50] As the gods have no body they have no experience. They are, therefore, in a position inferior to humans and cannot attain complete liberation. This idea explodes our fantasies of being god- and goddess-like, or of finding some kind of divine ideal in our partners. Contrary to popular misconceptions, yoga actually emphasizes the body as well as being *in* the experience of body. In Tantrism the dividing line between the divine and human worlds was a dotted

---

[49] Esther Myers, *Yoga & You*, p. 9.
[50] *Yoga: Immortality and Freedom*, p. 40.

one that could be crossed through systematic yoga practice.

We are never really able to separate from our body until the moment when the soul departs for the other world. Neither are we ever separated from the ground in this life. The goal is to bring the ego into a relationship of surrender to the Self without losing the ego altogether. Paradoxically, the ego must be strong enough to surrender. This statement is the foundation of an understanding of Jung's work. We must never lose consciousness in our relationship to the Self. Furthermore, we must never lose matter, our bodies, in our search for the transcendent. Over and over again, we touch the point where divine and human coincide. The newly created body in yoga and alchemy is the subtle body, the union of the opposites of psyche and matter. Practically speaking, this would mean that the insights gained in the mind are made real in the body. An insight is of no use if one is unable to utilize it. We must come into reality so that we can live in the world. The subtle body acts as intersector between these two worlds.

> Clearly, his [the yogin's] situation is paradoxical. For he is in life, and yet liberated; he has a body, and yet he knows himself and thereby is *purusa* (spirit); he lives in duration, yet at the same time shares in immortality; finally, he coincides with all Being, though he is but a fragment of it.[51]

Jung's studies on yoga were consistent with his research into alchemy, in that the goal of alchemy was the formation of the subtle body which is to be created through the art of making gold. The alchemical process is concerned with the cultivation of gold, in other words, with the development and increase of consciousness. Jung knew himself that alchemy was actually a Western form of practicing yoga and that alchemy valued the body as well as the feminine, both of which are renowned in Tantrism as representing a countermovement toward Christianity.[52] Both alchemy and yoga are concerned with the transformation of the body as the goal of the process. Yoga and the alchemical process are similar to active imagination, as trans-

---

[51] Ibid., p. 95.

[52] Sonu Shamdasani, *Introduction: Jung's Journey to the East*, in Jung, *The Psychology of Kundalini Yoga*, p. xlv.

formation in both of these instances is through the profound concentration of the imagination. A modern form of active imagination is a specific type of visualization where dream images, for example, can be implanted into various parts of the body allowing transformation to happen at the level of subtle body.[53] In yogic tradition, this model of concentration is what creates the world. Jung said once in a lecture that "it is not the world which produces concentration but concentration which produces the world."[54]

Ruth, forty years old, had suffered for a long time from such intense phobic anxieties that her life had become severely restricted. She came to analysis with the hope that bodywork might change something for her. She had tried various other therapies for years yet she felt little progress had been made. From the beginning I could sense a chilling emptiness in her; maternal warmth had been almost completely absent in her life. In addition to the phobias, she had suffered from sleep disturbances since she was a very young child and had virtually no help during those desperately lonely panic-ridden nights.

Once, near the beginning of our work together, I simply sat down next to her on the floor and placed my hands on her belly. So as not to be too intrusive, I had put a blanket over her and then placed my hands on top of the blanket. After I helped her get deeper into her breath in the belly, I moved to her feet. She told me later that she liked it very much when I had sat by her feet, and that during the deep breathing and relaxation she had seen colors behind her eyes—a big black circle with blue and red inside. She said these colors were moving all the time, as if they were floating on a beautiful pool of water. She experienced warm feelings inside.

When she got home she drew the image (Figure 4) because, she said, it helped her to keep the memory of these warm and calming colors with her throughout the week.

Ruth repeated to me that she feels the only connection she has to

---

[53] This is the work of "bodysoul rhythms" developed by Marion Woodman, Mary Hamilton and Ann Skinner in their 7-day intensive workshops for women.

[54] *Modern Psychology,* vol. 3, p. 15.

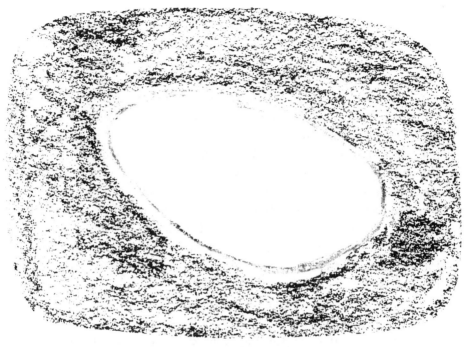

Figure 4. Analysand's drawing
(inner oval blue, surrounded by a red band; background black).

life and subsequently to relief from her acute panic attacks is through
bodywork. Her life feels black much of the time as expressed by the
black circle. During the bodywork experience, however, something
else began to emerge. From a deep place within her, a light blue center was constellated which was so calming for her that she felt she
could have achieved anything in that moment. Not long after this experience, Ruth was in fact able to attempt some of the activities she
feared most, such as riding a chair lift. Surrounding the blue in the
picture is red, the color of emotion and instinct. Within the blackness,
or *nigredo,* the opposite colors on the spectrum were constellated, that
is, the blue from the ultraviolet, or archetypal side, and the red from
the instinctual, or infrared side. Something in that short moment constellated and brought the two sides of spirit and instinct together. Ruth
had been held by the archetypal world. This experience was also aided

by my touch which, when given correctly, is always given from both the personal and the archetypal realms. As Eric Franklin tells us: "Touch is a powerful way to influence body image because it is one of the first ways we experience the boundary of the body."[55]

Going back to the essential problem of yoga for the West, we are reminded that Jung advised against Westerners' advocating the practice of yoga on the premise that we cannot understand *nirvana* without losing our hold on reality. Nevertheless, Jung led seminars on Kundalini yoga as well as on the visions of a woman, Christiana Morgan, whose journey is comparable to the ascent and descent of the Kundalini serpent. Always, Jung emphasizes the absolute necessity of having a relationship to the ground and to the body. The connection to the earth seems to be the essential point for Westerners, not merely for the sake of practicing yoga but also for its sake alone, as grounding is so sadly lacking in our culture today.

Eastern culture is introverted in contrast to that of the West. The mind of the Hindu, for example, simply takes for granted that the world was created from something inside, from a central energetic point. The Easterner already knows that the opposites are conceived as belonging to one and the same thing, that one can never actually separate heat from cold, yin from yang, and so on. They can more easily conceive, therefore, of a world that is free from conflict, as they will never lose the awareness of the opposites.

Consider what "freedom from the opposites" actually means. If one were really completely free of the opposites, one would be dead; there would be no more life at all. It is more correct, therefore, to say that the goal is rather to be able to *bear* the extremes of the opposites. In other words, to hold the stillness within until the vibration that exists between pairs of opposites comes to a halt, allowing the experience of ecstasy in the silence. This is what in yoga is termed *ekagrata*, which literally means "on a single point." *Ekagrata* puts an end to the fluctuation and dispersion of the states of consciousness.[56]

---

[55] *Dynamic Alignment Through Imagery*, p. 48.
[56] Eliade, *Yoga: Immortality and Freedom*, p. 55.

Jung writes in *The Visions Seminars* that consciousness in the East is already "down," that is, connected to the earth. It is logical, therefore, that in the East the goal is to connect to what is above, thereby compensating what is lacking; a clear awareness of consciousness does not exist in those who live closer to the unconscious. Jung says it is a mistake for those who live in the West to try to get higher and higher, as we are already living on too high a level, yearning only for the spirit world. We must seek rather to establish a relationship to our roots and to the unconscious. He further says that what is really needed is to establish the *connection* (my emphasis) between above and below.[57] This is the task of the *yogin* in our Western world.

As above, so below. The unconscious contains both aspects: the intellectual and spiritual as well as the dark and chthonic. June's lifelong desire to be a bird explains why she was sick. She was living in a fantasy world and, therefore, her connection to reality was minimal. Birds, as creatures of the air, are well-known symbols for the spirit. They also represent the head aspect of our being. June had lived life in her head, cut off from her body, thereby manifesting a thick, almost inhuman neck. It is worth mentioning here that Christiana Morgan had a vision in which something very strange happened. A white bird suddenly changed into a black hawk. This dark hawk swooped down to earth and came up again, but with an egg in its beak.[58]

We are reminded once again of the white plaster figures in June's initial dream. In this vision it becomes clear that the spirit not only represents a yearning for the light side, but has a dark aspect as well. June needed to integrate this dark aspect. In Morgan's vision the spirit is manifesting below in the dark, chthonic realm, as well as above in its aerial form. But the possibilities of a new beginning lie in the earthy aspect, the dark one, as the hawk brings the egg up out of the earth. We can see now that, along with the positive renewing aspects in the symbolism of the color white, June's initial dream pointed to a one-sidedness. As Marion Woodman explains, redemption does not come

---

[57] *The Visions Seminars*, p. 599.
[58] Ibid., p. 346.

about through searching for the light aspects of life:

> Yet rebirth to a higher level of consciousness is not accomplished by flying through the air. The ascent is balanced by the descent. The treasure is recovered through encountering the chthonic devourer, the dark side of the Great Mother. In Jung's terms, this is working at the deepest level of the somatic unconscious in order to bring to consciousness the subtle body.[59]

In the thirteenth century the Arabian alchemist, Avicenna, depicted an eagle flying high with a chain fastened onto its talons; the chain reaches down to the earth where a toad is fastened onto the other end. The verse that goes with it says:

> Bufonum terrenum Aquile conjunge volanti,
> In nostra cernes arte magisterium.[60]

—which translated means: "Connect the earthly toad with the flying eagle and thou shalt understand the secret of our art." (Figure 5)

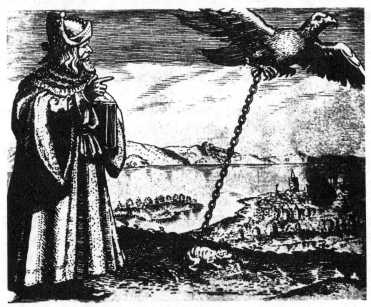

Figure 5. Flying eagle connected to a toad.

---

[59] Woodman and Dickson, *Dancing in the Flames*, p. 58.
[60] Quoted in Jung, *Nietzsche's* Zarathustra, p. 1413.

The eagle is a supreme example of the divine. It is the only animal that can look straight into the sun without becoming blind. Since it is solar and godlike, we are inflated if we identify with the eagle. The toad, on the other hand, has always been associated with the Earth Mother, especially in her function of helping at childbirth. The toad symbolized the uterus. There is a custom in some countries that if a woman has a disease of the uterus or some other kind of trouble relating to childbearing, rather than making a wax image of her uterus and hanging it in a church, she will make a wax image of a toad and suspend it near the statue of the Virgin.[61]

June's relation to the mother, to the womb, and, therefore, to her roots as a young woman, was lacking. In fact she had many dreams at the beginning of the analysis like this one:

I see a woman, unknown to me, who is pregnant. She was sharing a bed with a bad man. Then she went outside in the road and gave birth. Then she left the baby outside in the road while she went inside to wash herself. Later she went outside to see the child but I think that maybe she doesn't want the child but rather wants to get rid of it.

Here the mothering instinct is clearly missing. June was also unable to mother her inner child and thus have a relationship to her own body as well as to her feminine potential. Frogs and toads are a first attempt of nature toward making something like a human form, therefore they are symbols of human transformation. We see here that the toad element would bring what is lacking. Nietzsche thought of the frog as the inferior man living in the swamp or mire. Jung comments about Nietzsche's refusal to accept his instinctual side:

He refused to accept the other side because it was too repulsive, and because it became associated with a phobia: he suffered from the idea that he had to swallow a frog or a toad; whenever he saw one he had a compulsory inclination to swallow it. This appeared in a dream that a toad was sitting upon his hand; it referred to his syphilitic infection which he really could not accept, it was his clash with the earth, there the earth got him down.[62]

---

[61] Marie-Louise von Franz, *The Interpretation of Fairy Tales*, p. 73.
[62] *The Visions Seminars*, p. 543.

Frogs are green, the color of vegetation, hope and new life. Osiris's color was green, symbolizing resurrection. Frogs and toads live on the land but are dependent on water for life and, therefore, have a deep association to the unconscious. Mythologically, frogs and toads are the guardians of rain and they often play a part in incantations designed to bring rain in times of drought. Aymara Indians are said to make little images of frogs and other aquatic animals and place them on the tops of hills as a means of inducing rain. Some superstitions in Europe say that to kill a frog will cause rain to fall. In central India people will tie a frog to a rod covered with green leaves and branches of the *nim* tree and carry it from door to door singing:

> Send soon, O frog, the jewel of water!
> And ripen the wheat and millet in the field.[63]

We see clearly here that frogs and toads have a vital relationship to water, to the unconscious, and thus to the feminine, to the earth. They represent an essential element that is needed in order to balance the yearning for spirit in our time. They often appear in fairy tales as a bewitched form of a human figure, in order to bring about a redemption of the instinctual side of life.[64] As Jung says:

> I would mention the eagle and the toad ("the eagle flying through the air and the toad crawling on the ground") . . . the eagle representing Luna, "or Juno, Venus, Beya, who is fugitive and winged like the eagle, which flies up to the clouds and receives the rays of the sun in his eyes." The toad is the opposite of air, it is a contrary element, namely earth, whereon alone it moves by slow steps, and does not trust itself to another element. Its head is very heavy and gazes at the earth. For this reason it denotes philosophic earth, which cannot fly (i.e., cannot be sublimated), as it is firm and solid. Upon it as a foundation the golden house is to be built. Were it not for the earth in our work the air would fly away, neither would the fire have its nourishment, nor the water its vessel.[65]

Discovering a relationship to her body would bring June to the

---

[63] James Frazer, *The Golden Bough*, p. 72.
[64] See Marie-Louise von Franz, *Redemption Motifs in Fairy Tales*, p. 70.
[65] "The Components of the Coniunctio," *Mysterium Coniunctionis*, CW 14, par. 2.

place where a new structure was beginning to form inside herself, one which was based on having roots in the earth and in the world around her. In fact, something remarkable happened some months into the analysis. June had continued to mention now and again her desire to be a bird and simply escape the difficulties of earthly life. These statements usually occurred when her skin condition was at its worst. I knew then, especially at those times, that her connection to the positive feminine had been lost. Sometimes I suggested to her to move more slowly and pay attention to her feet when she was walking, so that she could feel some small orientation to her body, but she resisted my suggestions every time, saying that she would rather flit around like a bird. Since her childhood June had entertained this fantasy of being a bird, free and able to fly away into the heavens. She felt her life could then be perfect and carefree. Her life did indeed feel carefree, as she remembers it, until she was struck down by the skin disease at the age of twenty.

Some time later, when the skin condition began to improve, June told me that early one morning a bird had come to her window and had become trapped between the shutters and the window pane. It just stayed there and sang for hours until she got up and released it. June felt that the bird had been singing a message to her that she was now free. She knew immediately that she didn't need to be a bird anymore. She asked me again in the next hour whether or not we could begin some hands-on bodywork and I agreed. June knew that the time had come to begin to make a connection to the earth.

A few years later, when I was writing this text, I was hibernating in a magnificent old farmhouse nestled in the Alpilles in Provence, France. Very early one morning, before the sun had risen, I went to open the shutters on my study door. There, in the darkness, was a frog, quite large, sleeping between the door frame and the shutter. Unknowingly, in the darkness of the evening before, I had shut the frog in, displaying a marvelous synchronicity. Then I had no doubt that this work involves a deep and mysterious connection to the instinctual world.

4
The Spine As Axis Between Heaven and Earth

Come and see:
The world above and the world below are perfectly balanced:
Israel below, the angels above.
Of the angels it is written:
"He makes His angels spirits" (Psalm 104:4),
But when they descend, they put on the garments of this world.
If they did not put on a garment befitting this world
they could not endure in this world
and the world could not endure them.
—The Zohar.

My personal connection to bodywork is through the practice of yoga, which exemplifies the essence of connecting both to the earth below and to the sky above. It personifies the union of masculine and feminine through the union of opposites.

There are actually six schools of yoga but it is Hatha yoga, as well as breathing and meditation techniques, that we are most familiar with in the West. Hatha yoga was developed in order to give strength to the body through the poses (in Sanskrit they are called *asanas*). It emerged as a systematized way of doing yoga in the sixth century, and was practiced as a preparation for attaining higher consciousness. The advocates of Hatha yoga claimed that in order to purify the mind, it was first necessary for the body to undergo a process of purification. This philosophy corresponds directly to the alchemical process whereby the desired substance is first purified and then distilled out of the body, out of matter, so that it can later be reunited with the body in its purified form.

Hatha yoga is often mistakenly thought of as simply physical yoga, in other words, glorified physical exercise. The word *Hatha,* however, actually stands for *Ha,* meaning sun, and *tha,* moon. Hatha yoga therefore stands for the union of the masculine solar principle with the feminine lunar principle, being that the meaning of *yoga* is union. This union is desired in order to awaken higher consciousness. Jung compares the sun and the moon to the two eyes of heaven.[66] The aim of Hatha yoga is in fact the union of spirit *(prana)* and matter with the Self, the end-product being the divine immortal body. To my way of thinking, the aim of Hatha yoga is to develop the body into a strong yet flexible container that is able to hold the immense power of the spirit.

We often think that ecstatic, spiritual states only take place in the mind. As a matter of fact, however, mystical states can have a profound effect on the body, especially on the nervous system. A contemporary spiritual teacher, Da Free John, concluded that spiritual enlightenment must take place in the whole body. The goal, therefore, is to produce a divine body, or what is called in mysticism and alchemy a diamond body, the incorruptible breath-body which grows inside the flower of life. It was always the intention that immortality be attained through the transformation of the body. Being translucent as well as incorruptible, diamonds allow light to pass through unobstructed. Jung noted that in Chinese yoga the golden flower is the birthplace of the diamond body, which here is taken to mean the subtle body, the ethereal body.[67] Da Free John eloquently expresses the connection between religious experience and the body:

> The key to mystical language and religious metaphor is not theology or cosmology but anatomy. All the religious and cosmological language of mysticism is metaphorical. And the metaphors are symbols for anatomical features of the higher functional structures of the human individual.
>
> Those who enter deeply into the mystical dimension of experience soon discover that the cosmic design they expected to find in their inward path of ascent to God is in fact simply the design of their own anatomical or psycho-physical structures. Indeed, this is the secret divulged to initiates of mystical schools.[68]

---

[66] *The Visions Seminars*, p. 309.
[67] Ibid., p. 709.
[68] From *The Enlightenment of the Whole Body*, quoted in Georg Feuerstein, *Yoga: The Technology of Ecstasy*, p. 7.

Da Free John realized that first one must connect to reality through the body and then bring that experience inward. It is often after such an event that one begins the ascension into states of higher consciousness. Heaven and earth come together in ecstatic union.

One of the key figures in all of alchemy is Maria Prophetissa, a Jewish woman who lived in Egypt around the second or third century. A famous saying of hers is: "I am your earth and you are my sky."[69] Indeed, the sky is nothing without the earth, and vice versa. We find in Jung's *Psychology and Alchemy* an engraving attributed to Michael Maier in 1617 depicting the union of upper and lower (Figure 6).

Here Maria is pointing to a small mountain in the center of which is growing a white herb containing five branches. At the foot of this small mountain is an urn out of which rise two columns of smoke which then separate, forming a circle around the white herb that is ascending toward the top. These two columns in turn meet on their ascent two similar columns of smoke that are descending from an inverted urn situated in the heavenly realm. Everything above is the mirror image of that which is below. The commentary to the engraving reads in part:

Smoke loves smoke, and is loved by it in return:
But the white herb of the high mountain captures both.[70]

It is said that this white herb raises the bride of Mercurius, Philologia, to the level of her divine husband. She has been elevated to the immortal realm.[71] The whiteness of the herb signifies the possibility of new life, of healing in the eternal body. The *albedo* signals the coming of the new light after the long darkness of the night. According to the adepts, after this initial, difficult step has been taken the rest of the process becomes easier.

We see here, therefore, that the union of upper and lower, of the masculine with the feminine, and of the divine with the human worlds results in a five-branched white herb, each branch with a flower. This

---

[69] Source unknown.
[70] Raphael Patai, *The Jewish Alchemists*, p. 78.
[71] Jack Lindsay, *The Origins of Alchemy in Graeco-Roman Egypt*, p. 83.

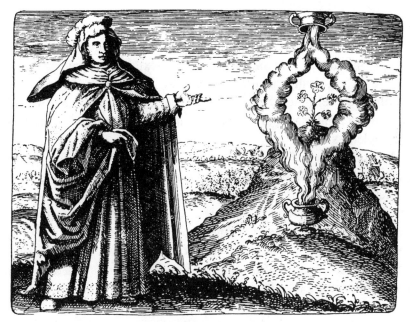

Figure 6. Maria Prophetissa.
In the background, the union of upper and lower.

flowering in the center of the whole process represents the elixir of life. The image of the white herb that sits in the center and connects the upper to the lower, and vice versa, in a continuous spiral motion, corresponds metaphorically to the function of the sacrum in our bodies. This large bone at the base of the spine connects the lower half of our body to the upper half. In fact, the sacrum acts as a pivotal center through which energy can flow.

The spine is the first structure that forms inside the womb, and all the other structures, such as the legs and arms, originate from the spine. The spine of a baby is soft and supple but as we age the spine often becomes stiff and inflexible. Many people "shrink" with the passing of time, partly because the body contains less and less water as it ages. Also, the body must be strong enough to resist gravity and to overcome the tendency to be pulled toward the earth's center. This demands strength as well as flexibility, for without flexibility strength only turns into rigidity. There is an ancient saying that was once told to me many years ago by an old yogi who lived in the hills above Tiberius in Israel: "You are as old as the flexibility of your spine." In fact, we do not really have to "age," we can in fact become more flexible and feel much healthier as we get older if we work with the spine in the right way and reeducate it in order to bring back its original suppleness.

The spine consists of individual vertebrae that form a four-curved structure. The smallest curve is found at the top and the largest and deepest is located at the bottom, in the sacral area. This sacrum, deepseated, curved and rounded, is essential to the structural design of the body, as it is a vital support for the spine. The fact that it is round ensures more stability at the base where it is needed.

Sitting at the bottom of the spine, the sacrum consists of five vertebrae that are fused together, making it ideal to both root and support the spinal column. The upper part of the sacrum is broader than the lumbar vertebrae that sit above it so that it can act as a weight-bearing structure. The sacrum becomes much shallower, however, as it continues down toward the coccyx, ending finally at the tail, which is assumed to be a remnant dating back to our ancestors.

June and I began our work with breathing back into the sacrum. This is done lying on one's back, most often with legs bent, as this position protects against injury to the lower back. It is important to note that for people with any kind of lower back discomfort at all, it is advisable never to lie on the floor with outstretched legs, especially at the beginning of the work.

We come once again to the breath. We remember that the *prima materia* symbolizes both the beginning and the end of the work. In the beginning, according to legend, Adam consisted of dust that had been gathered from the four corners of the world. However, Adam did not yet possess the gift of life:

> And the Lord God formed man of the dust of the ground, and breathed into his nostrils the breath of life; and man became a living soul.[72]

---

[72] Gen. 2:7.

Adam was only a lifeless statue before he received the breath of life. After he had been imbued with *prana*, the gift of life, Adam represented the lapis, or the final goal of the work. One of the earliest Greek alchemical treatises, the Book of Komarios, says:

> After the body had been hidden in the darkness, [the spirit] found it full of light. And the soul united with the body, since the body had become divine through its relation to the soul, and it dwelt in the soul. For the body clothed itself with the light of divinity, and the darkness departed from it, and all were united in love, body, soul, and spirit, and all became one; in this the mystery is hidden. But the mystery was fulfilled in their coming together, and the house was sealed, and the statue was erected, filled with light and divinity.[73]

Interestingly, Edward Edinger notes that nowadays we do not see many dreams in our practices that contain images of statues; instead people dream of dolls which are in fact contemporary images for the statue.[74] The statue stands for Adam in the lifeless state who is still in need of animation, still in need of the life force which enters the body through the breath.

At a crucial point in the analysis, just when June thought she might be ready to give up the image of being a bird and begin to do some bodywork with me, she had the following dream:

> We (me and other people) were in some sort of cave, we were building things, making things. I made a doll's head with blond hair. Then a lot of small birds came—blue ones, like the one who came to my window recently. A lot came, however, and it was difficult to get rid of them—they were all over me. They were clutching me. But we finally managed to get rid of them. They were in the room but I had the feeling of having them everywhere on my back. We ran away and kept shutting doors and windows from one room to another. Every time we tried to shut these doors and windows there would be a small hole in the window, or there was a key missing. We could never be really sure that the birds wouldn't come

---

[73] Quoted in Jung, "Adam and Eve," *Mysterium Coniunctionis*, CW 14, par. 559.
[74] *The Mysterium Lectures: A Journey through C.G. Jung's* Mysterium Coniunctionis, p. 234.

through so we had to shut all of them in. One man stayed at the last door inside. He said he would stay there because it ws safer and he could then make sure they wouldn't get out. Then I realized that I had forgotten my doll that I had made but I didn't go back because of the birds.

Being a bird for June had meant not confronting the shadow aspects and the dark side of life, the chthonic, the body. The birds here are contained in a cave, in the mother complex. June's lack of grounding in the positive mother forced her to fly away, looking for refuge in the spiritual realm. The body was then too weak to hold the spirit and she became sick. June had always wanted to be a bird but it had now become time for her to confront the dark aspects of life. June had actually suffered from intense depression before the onset of the neurodermatitis. As the psyche had not been strong enough to hold the conflict, the struggle went into her body where it could be seen. At the time of this dream, the skin disease had almost disappeared which brought up the former, almost immobilizing depression. At this point the analytic work became more difficult because, as noted earlier, it is much easier to see an illness in the body than to work with it in the psyche where it is relatively invisible.

In the dream June is trying to have a relationship with a doll, representing the shadow part in her that was being awakened, I believe for the first time, to the life force within her. This represented something completely untouched in her as in reality June is dark and doesn't have blond hair at all. The unconscious was attempting to bring life into her. In this dream one sees that the power of a complex will often become even stronger, making a last attempt to prove its autonomy, as it approaches consciousness. The birds are trying to prevent her from having a relationship with her new possibilities. Therefore, she must leave the doll behind. Yet at the end of the dream a helpful animus figure is able to protect her from the onslaught of the birds.[75]

---

[75] "Animus" is a term used by Jung to denote the masculine side of a woman. In its negative aspect, the animus is opinionated and judgmental and tries to dominate the woman's feminine side. In its most positive role, the animus represents her healing creative potential, mediating between her conscious mind and the unconscious.

The dream shows, however, that June is not yet ready to embrace her own life because in the dream she had to leave her doll behind. There were too many birds around which would ultimately divert her from her own work. We find this often in our work with people who are lacking a connection to reality—they become distracted by ungrounded spiritual pursuits. Nevertheless, the dream is hopeful as the energy is trying to move in the direction of developing a helpful animus that would ultimately bring her to her own creativity and fight for her own feminine. Here the unknown animus figure is able to keep the birds inside while June is able to escape to freedom, in spite of the fact that she has left the doll behind.

As June began to follow her own breath in a reclining position, I asked her first of all to simply observe her breath. This ability to witness what is happening is where consciousness begins. It is where we become the perceiver and the perceived at the same time. In the Mundaka Upanishad, III, 1, this is beautifully stated:

Like two golden birds perched on the selfsame tree,
Intimate friends, the ego and the Self
Dwell in the same body. The former eats
The sweet and sour fruits of the tree of life
While the latter looks on in detachment.[76]

We can also see here that the Self, representing a higher consciousness, stands behind every action taken by the ego. The ego serves as the instrument for the realization of the Self.

It is essential that in observing the breath one remains nonjudgmental. The breath may be tense and shallow, it may be fast, or it may be long, slow and relaxed. At the beginning of a breathing practice it is only necessary to observe what is happening with the breath, what is happening in the body. It is here that consciousness begins. With only the simple act of observation, the breath is able to change, to transform into a breath that not only quietens but also can go deeper, gradually penetrating the cells of the body where healing can

---

[76] *The Upanishads*, p. 115.

take place. Watching the breath allows for the body to begin to receive life, to feel the life-force within. The breath is our gift of life. It is the intelligence of the body.[77] It nourishes us into eternity. When we receive the breath, when we inhale, we need not make any effort, it will come in on its own. It is through trust that the incoming breath, the inhalation, will become relaxed and passive. If we do nothing, the breath will come in of its own accord. When we are relaxed, the lungs are free to receive the maximum amount of air available at this particular time. Some days there will be more accessible energy, some days less. It is vital that we remain detached during the inhalation in order to allow nature to take its course and for the full breath to evolve in itself.

I always begin with the breath centered in the belly, the *hara* center. Later one can move to other centers in the body. It is in the belly that we enter our prepsychological origins, mother, our development from the beginning of time. Ancient peoples believed that the emotional life was located in the belly and that thinking took place there or perhaps in the heart, but never in the head. The word *hara* literally means belly, which is the area below the navel, not the stomach as it is sometimes thought. The *hara* may be easily found by placing one's thumb on the navel and the fingers on the pubic bone below and allowing oneself to feel the breath moving in the area that lies between. The Japanese consider *hara* to be the center of gravity, therefore implying balance, a centering and a connection to the core of life. Concentration on the center constellates the life force par excellence.

It is with the exhalation, the out-breath, that we are able to eliminate impurities that are sitting in our bodies, causing all kinds of blockages, both psychic and physical. As we exhale, we empty the lungs as completely as possible so that the new breath, the prana, is able to come in with full capacity. When blockages are removed, the natural flow of energy can resume again and the body can release and let go. Approximately two thousand years ago, Patanjali described this mechanism wonderfully in Yoga Sutra 4.3:

---

[77] T.K.V. Desikachar, *The Heart of Yoga*, p. 22.

If a farmer wants to water his terraced fields, he does not have to carry the water in buckets to the various parts of his fields; he only has to open the retaining wall at the top. If he has laid out his terraces well and nothing blocks the flow of the water, it will be able to reach the last field and the furthest blade of grass without help from the farmer.[78]

The inhalation remains passive. One waits for the inhaling breath to come in its own time. The belly is filled with air, with life. One waits a moment, and then slowly the belly begins to expel the air. The exhalation has begun. All the work, either in a simple breathing exercise such as this one, or in the poses (*asanas*), is done on the exhaling breath. In order to exhale correctly, one must allow the entire weight of the body to rest back toward the spine. We relax back with the weight of gravity. The first mechanical obligation of the human structure is to satisfactorily meet the constant pull of gravity toward the center of the earth.[79] The back of the waist will gradually rest back on the floor. It may be easier to visualize the entire length of the back of the waist spreading out with the exhalation, as butter does when it begins to melt. Slowly more and more contact with the ground is made. One feels completely supported by the floor below such that no effort is needed to lie quietly. At first we seem able to take this awareness of support from the floor below for granted but, unfortunately, it is not so easy to give oneself over to anything, even to the floor below. It can take years for trust to enter the cells of the body. Yoga is not about performance and competition, it is about patience. It is about waiting until something begins to happen of its own accord.

The breath brings us to a state of quiet attention, the essence of yoga. As we follow the breath, the release and grounding of the exhalation balance the receptivity and expansion of the inhalation.[80] Keeping the above in mind, while lying on the floor we try to bring the awareness into the back of our bodies. I usually like to start lying on the floor as it is relatively easy to feel the spine on the floor in a

---

[78] Quoted in ibid., p. 58.
[79] Mabel Todd, *The Thinking Body*, p. 55.
[80] Esther Myers and Lynn Wylie, *The Ground, the Breath, & the Spine*, cover page.

reclining position. We are seldom connected to the back of our bodies. As we go forward everyday into the world we most often rely on the front of our bodies to give us an orientation. We have evolved more at the front of our bodies. The time has come to reverse our attention and bring the awareness into the back of the body. Our backs have simply followed along without our being aware of it. When we are working on the back of the body, we are working on the unconscious, as Jung tells us: "We have no eyes behind us; consequently "behind" is the region of the unseen, the unconscious."[81]

We go along in life with our backs remaining unconscious. With the commencement of this work, shadow aspects will begin to surface into consciousness for the first time, especially those aspects that relate to the negative mother complex. Our life seems to be going along just fine and then one day something just doesn't work anymore, we are in pain. It may seem very strange indeed; after all, we probably haven't actually *done* anything to our back, yet in distress it is screaming for attention. In our society it has now become essential that we begin to give attention to our body. If we look around us for a moment we will find people everywhere with back problems; we live a one-sided life when we neglect the back and the spine. We must undertake the immense task of connecting the dream world to the world of bodily reality. Jung explains very clearly in the following exchange the importance of combining bodywork with dream analysis:

> *Dr. Jung*: The Self is here leading the patient back to the tangible reality. You know in the psychology of the unconscious the body is always something like earth, it is heavy, dense, a thing which cannot be removed, an obstacle. It is the here and now, for to be really in the here and now, one must be in the body. But we have a peculiar faculty of stepping out of the body, which is again like the primitive. . . .

> *Miss Hannah*: How much would it help the patient if she should get back into her body? Would she be able to understand it or would she have to begin all over?

---

[81] "Individual Dream Symbolism in Relation to Alchemy," *Psychology and Alchemy*, CW 12, par. 55.

Dr. Jung: Anything experienced outside the body has the quality of being without body; so you must experience the whole thing over again, it must come in a new way. Then whatever you learn in analysis will happen to you in reality. It must be like that, because you are the point of identity, you are the one that experiences analysis and the one that experiences life. Whatever you experience outside of the body, in a dream for instance, is not experienced unless you take it into the body, because the body means the here and now. If you have a dream and let it pass by you, nothing has happened at all, even if it is the most amazing dream; but if you look at it with the purpose of trying to understand it, and succeed in understanding it, then you have taken it into the here and now, the body being a visible expression of the here and now. For instance, if you had not taken your body into this room, nobody would know you were here; though even if you seem to be in the body, it is by no means sure that you are, because your mind might be wandering without your realizing it. Then whatever is going on here would not be realized; it would be like a vague dream that floats in and out, and nothing has happened.[82]

What we are actually trying to do in this work is to develop vision from the back of the head. We do this by resting the back of the skull on the floor and, trying to follow the breath as it moves into the back of our body, we begin to get a wider and enlarged field of vision that is looking "backward." An added benefit is that our eyes will be able to rest. In this work, we are engaging in a relationship between the conscious and unconscious aspects of life. What is meant by neglecting the spine, therefore, is that it becomes dangerous solely by virtue of the fact that it has been neglected. Jung reminds us:

It would be wrong, however, to dwell only on the unfavourable side of the unconscious. In all ordinary cases the unconscious is unfavourable or dangerous only because we are not at one with it and therefore in opposition to it. A negative attitude to the unconscious, or its splitting off, is detrimental in so far as the dynamics of the unconscious are identical with instinctual energy. Disalliance with the unconscious is synonymous with loss of instinct and rootlessness.[83]

---

82 *The Visions Seminars*, p. 1316.
83 *Two Essays on Analytical Psychology*, CW 7, par. 195.

When we are not connected to our roots, we can either become sick in our bodies or experience terrible psychic problems such as intolerable anxiety or fear.

I am concentrating here on the center in the body which has been designated as the *hara* center, namely, the area which we more commonly know as the belly. There are other centers in the body that also deserve our attention, however, such as the heart chakra.[84] I find the belly to be the most useful center on which to focus, as it is through the belly, in the deepest recesses of our body, in the *muladhara* chakra, that we are able to root ourselves in the world.[85] The line of gravity passes through the center of the head down through the backs of the knees and ankles. The center of gravity can thus be measured as being inside the hip girdle at the level of the top of the sacrum, actually at the level of the fifth lumbar vertebra (the last vertebra in the spinal column before the sacrum). In other words, the center of gravity is a line that reaches from the center of the belly back to the top of the sacrum (Figure 7). Gravity brings us into contact with the spine.

Everything in the world has its own center, that place where the sacred manifests itself in totality. Many sources place the creation of man at the center of the world. It is said that God collected the dust from the four corners of the world and gathered it all together in the center of the earth where he created the first man, Adam.[86] Paradise was the "navel of the earth." According to Mesopotamian tradition, man was created at this navel, where there is the "link between Heaven and Earth."[87] Creation always takes place at a center. A Midrashic legend specifies that Adam was created in the city of Jerusalem. Also

---

[84] *Chakra* is a Sanskrit world meaning wheel or disk. A chakra is a point of intersection between various planes and is often described as a wheel-like spinning vortex. They are also called lotuses, symbolizing the unfolding of flower petals which metaphorically describe the opening of a chakra. Like lotuses, chakras have "petals" which symbolize a path of development from something primitive to the evolution of a greater consciousness.

[85] The *muladhara* chakra is discussed at length below, in chapt. 6.

[86] Zornberg, *Genesis: The Beginning of Desire,* p. 16.

[87] Mircea Eliade, *Images and Symbols,* pp. 43ff.

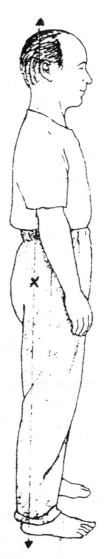

Figure 7. Standing with the force of gravity.

he was buried at the same spot where he was created, in Jerusalem, the center of the world.[88]

---

[88] Ibid.

Going back to the inhalation and the exhalation, we are trying to drop our weight into the floor so that the sacrum makes more and more contact with the floor with each breath. No movement or change is possible without the awareness of the breath. Breath is the transformer. An attempt to change the structure of the body without bringing in an awareness of the breath will only result in a kind of forcing, a forcing which is only connected to willpower and which in the end has nothing to do with deep transformation. With each exhalation we bring more and more energy into the sacral area. A warming of the area begins to take place, simply by allowing the breath to penetrate. Warmth is nourishment that comes from the positive mother, and as one drops more and more into the sacrum the spine in turn begins to drop back into the floor, and one begins to feel held by the floor below, by the earth, by the Great Mother.

As already mentioned, the breath in the belly is being directed down toward the base of the spine. It is a surprise for us when we learn that the actual depth of the spine takes up approximately half of the distance between the front and the back of the body. I try to have my yoga students visualize the breath coming down as far as the front of the spine in the center of the body at the end of the exhalation. This is a very gradual process, however, and it requires time and patience for the breath to enter the body on such a deep level.

June began to experience a center within her own body after the first session of yoga that we did together. That night she dreamt the following:

> Somebody gave me different insects—beetles and spiders. I wasn't scared.
> They were small ones. I covered them with a blue plastic basket so that
> they couldn't crawl away. I was confused why somebody would give you
> insects but somehow I knew that I had to look after them.

In this context, insects signify basic dissociated elements. June had in fact been quite dissociated, especially from her body. Here she is able to bring the dissociated elements together, to begin the task of unifying what had previously been fragmented.

Something had profoundly changed. Through the bodywork, June was beginning to approach the problem of looking after the insects in a careful, conscious way. As insects exist at a purely instinctual level, this dream was an excellent indication for June to begin to relate to her instinctual side, to her body. The two sides of the spectrum were coming into balance. June associated the plastic basket to a red one that she loved and used as a child when she went to ballet classes. This time the ballet basket is blue, however, suggesting a connection to the world of the spirits. Here the spirit contains the raw instinctual life. To be with insects means to be in contact with something very simple, the beginnings of life, also something deep in the unconscious. The basket provides the container for the dissociation. Ballet is also a form of bodywork that involves the spine.

The energy is slowly gathering into the sacrum with each exhaling breath as it drops back into the floor. The breath continues to open and release the sacrum as well as the muscles and bones that surround it. The word *sacrum* comes originally from the Latin word *sacer,* meaning "holy" or "sacred." The center of gravity is located at the top of the sacrum, which thus makes the sacrum the focal point of our relationship to the ground, to the body, and to our human reality. *Hara* is the seat of all instinctual and psychic life:

> *Hara* implies for the Japanese all that he considers essential to man's character and destiny. *Hara* is the center of the human body—but the body, because it is a human body, is more than a biological-physiological entity. It is at the same time the center in a spiritual sense or, to be more accurate, a nature-given spiritual sense.[89]

Hara, then, represents one's center, the center always implying something sacred, the area of absolute reality.

Bringing energy into the sacrum connects us to the archetypal reality of everlasting time. We remember that the sacrum consists of five bones fused together forming a strong, curved structure that supports the spine. The fact that the sacrum is made up of five bones is no coincidence. Five signifies the number of the human being; we have five

---

[89] Karl von Durkheim, *Hara: The Vital Center of Man,* p. 49.

senses, five fingers, and five toes. The number five, therefore, represents a totality in a concrete, material, body way.

The so-called Axiom of Maria further clarifies the meaning of the number five:

> One becomes two, two becomes three, and out of the third comes the one as the fourth.[90]

If we consider the movement from two to three (one is not considered to be a number in mathematics as nothing precedes it and, therefore, it does not "count"), we find that three comes out of a resolution of the conflict implied in the number two. Three, therefore, represents a unity, a *one*, so to speak, that comes out of the number two. Three actually leads us back to the primal number, to the number one. In fact all numbers will lead us back to the one. Two things are thus happening simultaneously: the numbers are progressing from one to infinity and at the same time they are proceeding in a retrograde manner, always leading us back to the one. In this way the number three, which we have already identified as a unitary number, becomes the number four. The number four, therefore, does not originate through progression from the preceding number three, but was always in existence from the beginning.[91] The relationship of the four to the one is depicted in a modern Navaho Indian drawing (Figure 8).

We see here that there are four heads, therefore four goddesses. Upon careful observation, however, we see that the series actually begins with the skirt of the fourth goddess, making the one and the four identical and containing the other three figures. The original one is as the number four. Four leads us back to the original unity, to the *unus mundus*.[92]

The progression from four to five happens in a similar manner: five represents the unity within the number four. In China the number five holds the same meaning as four does in Western culture, as five is

---

[90] Quoted in "Introduction to the Religious and Psychological Problems of Alchemy," *Psychology and Alchemy*, CW 12, par. 26.
[91] See Marie-Louise von Franz, *Number and Time*, p. 64.
[92] Ibid., p. 130.

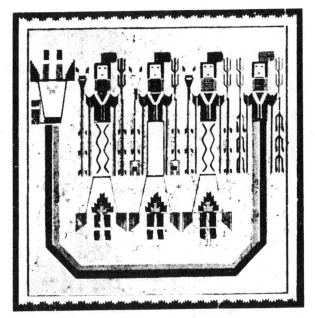

Figure 8. Handicraft tile of the Tama Indian settlement.

taken there to be the center of the four. Five is the *quinta essentia*, the essence, the kernel in the center of the four:[93]

Five is where four becomes a reality; five is the number of the natural man, not the ideal man. Nature does not omit the bodily aspect in the number five. Rupescissa, a Jewish alchemist of the fourteenth century, wrote of the *quinta essentia* as being the connection between the divine and the human world:

> This fifth essence is the human heaven which the Most High created for the conservation of the four qualities of the human body, just as [He created] the heaven for the conservation of the whole universe.[94]

---

[93] Ibid., pp. 120f.
[94] Quoted in Patai, *The Jewish Alchemists*, p. 205.

Within the circle of totality there is contained a central point of consciousness, the number five as the center of the totality of the four, five as the ego, as the center of consciousness; the ego in the center brings reality to the irrational four. Five, embodying the human being, represents the earth in all her aspects (Figure 9). As Jung says,

> Earth occupies the central position as the fifth element, though it is not the quintessence and goal of the work but rather its basis, corresponding to terra as the arcane substance in Western alchemy.[95]

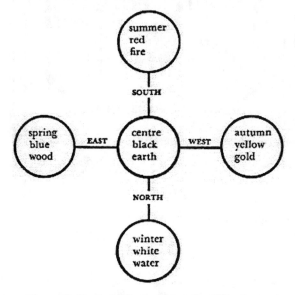

Figure 9. Earth in the center as the fifth element.

When we come to the center, we reach the eternal within. The energy within this central point is manifested in the archetypal urge to become who one is, who one is meant by Nature to become. All that is contained within this center Jung called the Self, the totality of everything contained within the psyche. This totality includes the conscious world, the personal unconscious, and the collective unconscious which

---

[95] "The Personification of the Opposites," *Mysterium Coniunctionis*, CW 14, par. 249.

comprises the universal, indestructible archetypal world.

The sacrum as sacred or "holy bone," as we have called it, is the center of the divine body. The center of gravity is located at its apex; the sacrum forms the base of the long curved structure at the back of our body, the spine. The first thing that mankind did in ancient times was to draw a straight vertical line connecting the earth with the heavens. This line became their focal point of orientation. For the Hindus, this line later became the idea of a mountain containing the axis around which the world turns, paradoxically motionless but in constant motion. Mountains are often regarded as the place where the sky and the earth come together in a central point, through which travels the *axis mundi,* the pillar that supports the world.

God, being the center of the universe, created man in his likeness, thus man, as microcosm, represents the center of the world, containing all within himself alone. Inner and outer collectively form the totality:

> Man is to be esteemed a little world, and in all respects he is to be compared to a world. The bones under his skin are likened to mountains, for by them is the body strengthened, even as the earth is by rocks, and the flesh is taken for earth, and the great blood vessels for great rivers, and the little ones for small streams that pour into the great rivers. The bladder is the sea, wherein the great as well as the small streams congregate. The hair is compared to sprouting herbs, the nails on the hands and feet, and whatever else may be discovered inside and outside a man, all according to its kind is compared to the world.[96]

Man as microcosm is illustrated in Figure 10, where we see the Hindu god Krsna embodying the entire universe within himself. As it says in the Taittiriya Upanishad 1:7:

> Earth, sky, worlds above, quarters and their halves;
> Fire, air, sun, moon, and stars; water, herbs, trees,
> Space, and entity are the elements.
> Eye, ear, mind, tongue, and touch; skin, flesh, muscle,
> Marrow, and skeleton; and the five
> Vital forces constitute the body.

---

[96] "The Visions of Zosimos," *Alchemical Studies*, CW 13, par. 122

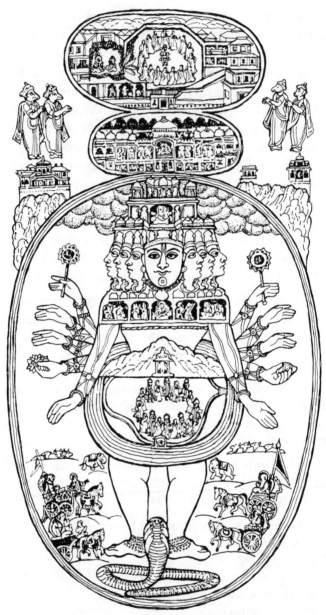

Figure 10. The cosmic Krsna, showing earth (in the region of his stomach) and the heavens at the top, both with their (earthly and eternal) round dances.

The sage, contemplating these sets of five,
Discovered that everything is holy.
Man can complete the inner with the outer.

Another illustration (Figure 11) shows in detail the earth segment within the macrocosm. In the center of the earth stands the gigantic mountain of Meru, which is said to prop up the heavens many millions of feet above. Mountains connect the lower world with the upper one, they unite heaven and earth, and they intersect the divine with the human world.

Caves that were directly adjacent to mountains became the birthplace of many of the Greek gods. In fact several heroes, Achilles for example, were born or raised on a mountain. Esoterically, the image of a mountain depicts the body seated motionless in meditation. Seen

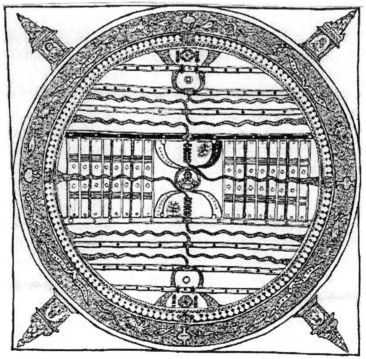

Figure 11. Map of the central portion of earth.

in this way, the body appears as a triangle, in a kind of peaked shape, akin to a mountain. The Buddhists describe the body in meditation as being Mount Meru, the center of their world and identified with the spine.

Mount Meru, being at the center of the universe, implies a stillness within. This is one of the most important goals of yoga: to bring the body and mind into stillness so that one can experience the inner world. Concentration and utter discipline are needed in order to enter and to remain in the center. The unconscious actually moves continuously, circumambulating a center, and as the center becomes closer, it becomes more and more distinct. In a miraculous way, the center acts as a kind of magnet on the surrounding incompatible and chaotic material, gradually drawing these contents closer in order that an image of man may force its way through the manifesting chaos. It is as though the center is actually being fertilized by the creative contents of the unconscious. In this way, creativity manifests itself. Wondrously, a kind of mystical circle forms around the center, around the core we call the Self, serving as a protection from the outside world and allowing what is inside to further intensify. In Tantric yoga the highest achievement is esteemed to be the production of such a center, which when concentrated upon will strengthen the container of its own accord.

The image of complete stillness is illustrated in the *I Ching,* hexagram 52, "Keeping Still, Mountain." In the upper trigram we find the male principle striving upward, and in the lower, identical doubled trigram we find the feminine principle descending. Both movements are equal which means that there is no longer motion, everything has come to a complete rest. There is actually a division in the middle of the hexagram which allows for the upper trigram to move upward and for the bottom one to proceed downwards. Rigidity is overcome through allowing the emergence of the opposites. In his commentary Richard Wilhelm adds: "Possibly the words of the text embody directions for the practice of yoga."[97]

---

[97] *The I Ching or Book of Changes,* p. 201.

In various Hatha yoga writings, the spine, being the axis around which the energies in the body revolve, is likened to a mountain in the macrocosm. *Tadasana* in Sanskrit is translated as "mountain" and is the name for the basic standing pose in yoga. It is the simplest pose, yet it is also the hardest to do correctly. The ability to stand absolutely straight while preserving inner stability is the goal of all the poses that we do. *Tadasana*, or *tad-asana*, meaning mountain pose, has as its root the word *asana*, which has as its root *as*, meaning "to stay," "to be," or "to sit." *Asana* itself translates as "posture," meaning that we strive just "to be" in a pose; in other words, ideally we would approach each pose with a steadiness and security that come from a place deep within us that connects to that which is essential. When we stop trying to "do" the poses, that is when the ecstatic moment of true stillness will come.

Mircea Eliade explicitly states that in order to achieve ultimate stillness, the *asanas* must be done with absolute concentration:

> On the plane of the "body," *asana* is an *ekagrata*, a concentration on a single point; the body is "tensed," concentrated in a single position. Just as *ekagrata* puts an end to the fluctuation and dispersion of the states of consciousness, so *asana* puts an end to the mobility and disposability of the body, by reducing the infinity of possible positions to a single archetypal, iconographic posture. We shall soon see that the tendency toward "unification" and "totalization" is a feature of all yogic techniques.[98]

In *tadasana* we stand as a mountain, in other words, with a huge firm base beneath our feet. At the same time, in the upper body we are striving to achieve a feeling of expansiveness, while constantly maintaining a position of utter stillness. The mountain symbolizes stability and a cessation of motion which is the beginning and the end of all our movements, as the *prima materia* is the initial point as well as the end-goal. In fact, all the other *asanas* that we do are a variation of *tadasana*. The body itself is just unstable enough for there to exist a constant struggle for equilibrium between its parts. In *tadasana* we experience this at its fullest.

---

[98] *Yoga, The Technology of Ecstasy*, p. 54.

In *tadasana* we grow roots into the floor. Actually we grow roots down past the floor we are standing on; we grow them through the floor to the earth below, and we continue growing the roots until they reach the center of the earth. The deeper we are able to drop down, the deeper the descent into the unconscious. Many of us are unconnected to a life force that is able to sustain us in moments of darkness and chaos. This force, or what an alchemist termed the "global fire," is found in the center of the earth. For with the darkness from below will come the light from above. When we become connected to this sacred place at the core of the earth, true healing can take place. It is the center of the earth that contains the archetypes, the central nucleus where healing becomes possible.

We have become unstable for various reasons. Today it seems that we are without roots, without a genuine connection to where we have come from, to where we are in the moment, and to where we are headed in the future. Allowing ourselves to connect to the deep-seated origins that existed thousands of years before us brings healing at a profound mystical level.

We actually drop roots from the waist downward, allowing the force of gravity to pull us. It is as if a magnet were actually drawing us into the floor. The world of the archetypes is a magnetic one; it pulls us in with tremendous force, yet we must resist being just sucked in, in order to avoid possession or, in the worst circumstances, psychosis. It is similar to the force of gravity, the power that pulls us toward the earth, which is balanced by an equal resistance to gravity, a pull in the opposite direction. Gravity is counteracted by the tendency of living things to expand and grow upward toward the sun. When there is too much energy manifesting on one side, at some point the energy must turn into its opposite. Thus, as we exert pressure downward, there will come an equal opposing thrust upward. It is crucial that, as we come up after dropping down well into our heels, we do not simply leave our feet altogether and continue upward but that we keep the connection to what is below as our bodies stretch upward toward the heavens. There is no such thing as a force acting alone. Our own muscles have to counteract each other in order to cause movement.

We find in the body, therefore, that a downward force always complies with the gravitational force while at the same time an opposition to the pull of gravity allows us to stand upright on the ground. The body adores the feeling of energy traveling through our limbs, yearning for more and more extension. The closer we are to the center within, the less expenditure of energy will be required to maintain an equilibrium, thereby allowing the maximum possible energy for healing to take place. What matters is the amount of energy we have at our disposal, as without it inertia will result. Gradually, if *tadasana* is maintained correctly, a whole new attitude to the body develops, bringing a greater overall energy out of the reconciliation of these universal opposites. A calmness will result, which is the genuine meaning of "mountain."

When we go down, so to speak, we begin to enter the realm of the collective unconscious, at a very archaic level where nature exists in her purest form. There we find the hope for a renewed life. Jung says:

> Going down to the collective level always means going back in time. . . .
> It is a regressive progress, one could say, but the more she [Christiana Morgan] goes back in time, the more time comes to meet her. It is as if she were approaching a mirror, and the nearer she approaches it, the nearer comes the image in the mirror.[99]

When we do approach our distant past, we touch not only the collective unconscious but also our own personal beginnings. We are touching all the unfulfilled lives that came before us and we are redeeming them, living them out, so to speak, thereby preparing the way ahead for the next generation. The more we are able to drop down, the more the spine can elongate, the more our spine comes into alignment with the *axis mundi,* the center of the earth. Proper alignment is always a balance between sufficient muscular activity to create an upright posture and sufficient relaxation for this stance to be as effortless as possible. We are then brought into relationship with the positive, cherishing Great Mother who will resonate at the deepest layers in the cells of our body. Through relating to this archetype, we

---

[99] *The Visions Seminars*, pp. 59ff.

discover the miracle of creativity.

Tadasana implies the separation of the opposites out of a disordered world. In the initial stages of bodywork, specifically the work on the spine, one usually encounters a chaotic mess which may manifest in different forms. For example, a body that may appear flexible and supple may actually contain many very tight and inflexible parts, while paradoxically a tight body may actually be able to do "more" in the beginning, being held up by its own rigidity. Normally one encounters a spine that has shortened through stress as well as the normal aging process. As a result, the spinal structure does not flow in a congruous way when in motion. The elongation of the spine is one of the most important ways in which we create an "immortal body," one which is able to resist the temptations of time to become weary, inflexible and shorter. In this case "shorter" often includes a lower self esteem, brought on partially by the physical changes in the body itself and partially by the feeling of many people that they have not lived, a feeling of resentment at their bodies for becoming less capable as they age. The work of constantly elongating the spine brings about a tremendous sense of being alive, often experienced for the first time.

The feeling of being alive is deeply connected to the life force. Nancy came into analysis knowing that something was wrong in her life but she had no idea what it could be. She comes from a family where feeling was essentially missing. An immobilizing fear had taken over her life. After three years of analysis Nancy dreamt:

> A man, a kind of Guru figure or some other kind of authority I'm not sure what, is sitting on my neck. I am kneeling or sitting and my head is between his legs. I feel his weight pushing down so heavily on me that my movements are almost completely restricted. I actually wake up from the dream with pain in my shoulders and neck.
>
> A woman comes in and presses on a vertebra at the base of my spine and says: "We must stretch and elongate the spine." But the man says, no, we must bend it. She repeats: "Stretch and elongate."

Beneath a terrible paralyzing animus possession, Nancy is beginning to find her connection to the feminine. In reality she is quite bent over, suffering from the beginnings of osteoporosis at the early age of thirty-eight. She has literally been weighed down by life, the constant pressure to meet the expectations of others. The flow of life, which in a natural course of events would move through the spine, has been inhibited by a huge fear of contact with her instinctual life and all its related, pent-up feelings of grief and rage. Just the possibility of such a contact has brought her closer to a primal fear of annihilation.

In body language, we can think of this potential to experience life as resting in the spinal column itself, the backbone of life. Nancy has gradually been able to let the spine go in our sessions together and is discovering movement and spontaneity for the first time. In the above dream we begin to see the transformation incorporated through the feminine shadow figure who is moving her away from god-like animus projections that hinder life. This dream illustrates how possession by the negative animus can lead to a woman's body problems and that it is the feminine that must redeem her. Marie-Louise von Franz used to say that when she had pains in her neck and shoulder area, she knew that she had been in the animus.[100]

When the spine lengthens to its natural state, the axis of heaven and earth is constellated. In Talmudic legend, it is said that although the heavens and the earth contain entirely different elements, they were nevertheless created as a unit, "like the pot and its cover." The only distinct act of separation during creation was on the second day when the upper waters were separated from the lower ones. It is on this second day that God omitted to say that all was good. Separation must entail suffering as the opposites move apart. We can almost hear the groaning of the universe during the act of separation. It is said that all other acts during creation were unifying ones.[101] It is as if we find ourselves at the beginning of the work back in the chaos of the waters of the beginnings of life, back at the *nigredo,* before the creation of consciousness. When we are overcome by such disorder and confusion, we are unable either to stand still or to move forward, but are in-

---

[100] I am grateful to Dr. Hermann Strobel for this anecdote.
[101] Louis Ginzberg, *Legends of the Bible,* pp. 3ff.

stead propelled back into chaos. Out of this condition the upper must be separated from the lower. Division into two is essential in order to bring what has been *in potentia* into reality; we must bring matter to consciousness.

Jung describes the condition of *unio mentalis* where one steps away from the body in order to engender objective insights, but it is in the *unio corporalis* that we are able to bring these insights back into the body and where we encounter the subtle body in its glorious resonance. As Jung says: "Its reality is merely potential and is validated only by a union with the physical world of the body."[102]

The spine may be thought of as being divided into two distinct parts in order to bring the body to consciousness. The method can be described as follows: Standing in *tadasana*, we feel the weight of the body being pulled down by gravity. The weight should be placed as evenly as possible on both feet, so that imaginally one could paint the soles of the feet with black ink and upon moving away from the spot where we are standing, two beautifully uniform imprints will remain. This of course is an idealized image, nevertheless it remains important to hold this image within while standing firmly on both feet. It is said in the Talmud that even after one has finished praying, if one has not physically moved one's feet, then one is still standing in the presence of God.

On an exhalation, we breathe down into the heels. Each *asana* has its specific roots which go down into the earth and hold us there firmly; when we are standing these roots become our heels. It should be remembered that we are trying to reconnect to the center of the earth through breathing down into the heels. When we go into ground, we enter body, the holy place where God is incarnated within us. If we are not afraid of life, then we will be able to stand back on our heels without the fear of falling backward. We will know that God is always standing behind us through the relationship to the unconscious.

The more we are able to breathe down into the heels, the more the upper body will be free to stretch and release upward. The spine actu-

---

[102] "The Conjunction," *Mysterium Coniunctionis*, CW 14, par. 664.

ally divides in order to make this possible. We remember the story of Phan-Ku who separated earth and heaven by thirty thousand miles in order to create space for himself.[103] The creation of space is what allows something new to happen. It is fundamental that our heels become our anchor that will then allow the spine to stretch away from its root, the sacrum. Vanda Scaravelli has called this movement a "wave" and in an interview with Esther Myers and Kim Echlin, she explains how the natural pull of gravity leads into the "wave" in the spine:

> It's about the way the spine moves from the heels to the top of the head with gravity. You let the body sink, sink, sink, and the upper part becomes light. The more you sink, the more the upper part becomes light and there is a beautiful wave in the body, and the body moves with the wave. The wave to the ground allows the gravity in the spine and through the spine, and energy goes through the top of the head. The body is pulled down, and from the waist up there is a wonderful way of feeling, of behaving, of moving. It gives a sense of authority, of freedom, of beauty.[104]

The spine divides at the level of the waist. Striving toward consciousness brings about the separation of the opposites. Simply put, from the waist down the body is pulled downward by gravity, and from the waist upward the upper body elongates and stretches up toward the heavens. Upon careful anatomical investigation, however, one finds that the spine does not actually divide at the sacrum but rather at the fifth lumbar vertebra, the vertebra which lies just above and connects to the sacrum (Figure 12).

Here again is the number five, the *quinta essentia.* There are five lumbar vertebrae that sit above the sacrum, which we remember also consists of five vertebrae fused together to make one unit. The energy seems to concentrate itself specifically in the area of this last, the fifth lumbar vertebra. L5 is the place in the spine that intersects the twenty-four single vertebrae and the sacrum. This exact spot which lies directly above and is also connected to the sacrum, is the *quinta essentia,* the place of division and transformation in the spine, and, conse-

---

[103] See above, p. 15.
[104] "Awakening the Spine," in *Yoga Journal,* June 1996, pp. 70f.

quently, in the entire body, for the spine is our backbone, supporting us from behind, as does the unconscious.

We are in the zone of the sacred, the place of something unknown and mysterious that opposes chaos and death. Sacredness implies a sense of a greater being existing separate from and outside of oneself, something "numinous,"[105] a mystical experience. Hindu writings tell

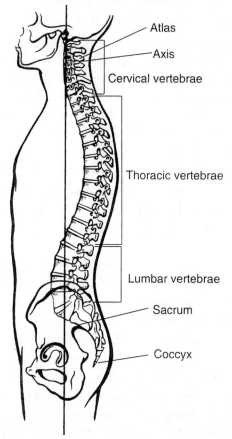

Atlas

Axis

Cervical vertebrae

Thoracic vertebrae

Lumbar vertebrae

Sacrum

Coccyx

Figure 12. The vertebral column consists of 24 separate vertebrae, composite vertebrae, the sacrum and the coccyx.

---

[105] Numinosity, a term coined by the German theologian Rudolph Otto, is characterized by a feeling of awe, fascination and mystery.

us that something becomes sacred whenever our attention is directed to it in a special way. The sacrum has been thought of as the "holy bone" for centuries; as matter, it acts as transformer to the eternal world. It is holy because on it rests the eternal bone, the fifth lumbar vertebra.

A Midrashic legend identifies an indestructible bone at the base of the spinal column called *luz*, shaped like an almond and around which a new body will be formed during the resurrection of the dead in the Messianic Age. This bone is said to survive the disintegration of the body after burial, the only part of the body that will not disintegrate with time. Evidence of this is given in the Vayikra Rabbah 18:1:

> As proof, Rabbi Yehoshua placed a *luz* in water, and it did not dissolve; he let it pass through the millstones, but it was not ground; he put it in a fire, but it was not incinerated; he placed it on an anvil and struck it with a hammer; the anvil was flattened out and the hammer split, but the *luz* remained undamaged.[106]

During the resurrection, the revivifying agent will be the dew made of the light that was present when God created the world but which has been concealed ever since. It is said that even those bodies which have decomposed will be reconstructed from the *luz* bone in their spine. Legend tells us that those who bow to God are thought to guarantee themselves a resurrected body because they stimulate the *luz* bone when they bend their spine in prayer.

Dew is a transformer, vital to life; its absence causes a drought, so its presence is a matter of life and death for farmers. We are told in the Zohar that "dew wakens the dead and is the food of the holy."[107] It is said that the manna which appeared in the wilderness after the exodus from Egypt was covered both above and below with white dew. It was the dew that miraculously revived the Israelites when they had died of fright at Mount Sinai after hearing the voice of God.[108] The dew purifies and vivifies the body, enabling it to receive the soul, which, as it

---

[106] Avraham Yaakov Finkel, *In My Flesh I See God*, p. 179.
[107] Quoted in "The Conjunction," *Mysterium Coniunctionis*, CW 14, par. 701n.
[108] Alan Unterman, *Dictionary of Jewish Lore and Legend*, p. 62.

descends from heaven toward incarnation, appears identical to the dew falling from heaven. The tears that Isis wept as she gathered together the scattered limbs of Osiris were the transforming agent that brought her beloved back to life.

The moisture contained in the dew is the alchemical divine water, the elixir of immortality. We are born into the eternal womb which contains the water of life. Water is the basic material of life, the *prima materia*, whence we came and whither we shall return. The potential of transformation through the connection to the fifth lumbar vertebra, the *luz* bone, is made possible through its connection to the divine water, the dew which wakens the dead out of their sleep and brings consciousness, for, as Jung says:

> The falling dew signals resuscitation and a new light: the ever deeper descent into the unconscious suddenly becomes illumination from above. For, when the soul vanished at death, it was not lost; in that other world it formed the living counterpole to the state of death in this world. Its reappearance from above is already indicated by the dewy moisture . . . . while on the other hand dew is synonymous with the *aqua permanens*, the *aqua sapientiae*, which in turn signifies illumination through the realization of meaning.[109]

As one persists with this work, one becomes more and more conscious of the energy intensifying and gathering in this relatively small area at the top of and just above the sacrum. And as one comes closer to the innermost center, a renewal of the personality becomes possible. This center serves as container, the vessel of rebirth which is continually being fertilized by the heavenly water, the dew of transformation.

Luz is often called by another name—Jerusalem, denoting the center of the world and the holiest of cities. A famous passage in Midrash Tanhima speaks to the meaning of the sacred city:

> Just as the navel is found at the center of a human being, so the land of Israel is found at the center of the world. Jerusalem is at the center of the land of Israel, and the temple is at the center of Jerusalem, the Holy of

---

[109] "The Psychology of the Transference," *The Practice of Psychotherapy*, CW 16, par. 493.

Holies is at the center of the temple, the Ark is at the center of the Holy of Holies, and the Foundation Stone is in front of the Ark, which spot is the foundation of the world.[110]

In ancient Israel, this Foundation Stone played the same role as did the primordial earth in Egypt: it was the first solid material to emerge from the waters of creation; it was also upon this stone that the world was created. Jung called Jerusalem the white city, the city of enlightenment, the promised land on the mountain of Meru.[111] In the Midrash it is also said that Adam, as *prima materia*, was fashioned in Jerusalem, Jerusalem being the center of the indestructible and everlasting world. Consciousness is created in the center where the opposites separate.

Let us return to the vertical separation of the spine into two parts, upper and lower; the upper as heaven is represented by the crown of the head while the lower as earth is embodied by the lower part of the spine, the sacrum, the root chakra. We in fact dismember the spine into two segments, initially allowing them to function independently. Heaven and earth must be broken apart in order that they may one day come together again in a new way, unburdened, as a new light is born out of the darkness. Only in this way can our neurotic symptoms and illnesses make way for a new consciousness that must embrace psyche and soma as one.

Another way of looking at the separation of the spine is to see that the two parts fit together in a remarkable way. In his commentary on the origin of the sacred Chinese book, *The Secret of the Golden Flower*, Richard Wilhelm tells us that the words "Golden Flower" in Chinese actually include the word "light." It is our task to bring transforming light into the body. He explains further:

If one writes the two characters one above the other, so that they touch, the lower part of the upper character and the upper part of the lower character make the character for "light" (*kuang*).[112]

---

[110] Quoted in John Lundquist, *The Temple: Meeting Place of Heaven and Earth*, p. 7.

[111] *The Vision Seminars*, p. 721.

[112] *The Secret of the Golden Flower*, p. 9.

In other words, when written vertically the two characters fit together perfectly to create a new word, "light," akin to the functioning of the two separated parts of the spine. Both sections must function on their own but each is indispensable for the proper functioning of the other. The upper spine can be thought of as mind or spirit, the lower spine as instinct or body, therefore closer to the earthly realm. We have here an example of an exquisite reciprocal working relationship, as we also have in the reciprocity between psyche and soma.

In the "wave" we go down in order to go up. It sounds simple but actually finding ground is often extremely difficult, especially in our culture where we have lost the connection to our origins. In other words, we begin by finding grounding from below, through the connection of our feet to the earth. We are reborn through coming into our feet. According to a hymn from the Rg Veda,[113] men were born from the feet of the god Purusa.[114] It is with the feet that we have our standpoint in life. Thus we become aware of desire and of the essence of what we are becoming in the experience of knowing solid ground. One might ask why we first go down through the heels before going up, rather than the reverse. Jung answers the question simply:

> We can explain a house not only from the attic downwards, but from the basement upwards, and the latter explanation has the prime advantage of being genetically the more correct, since houses are in fact built bottomside first, and the beginning of all things is simple and crude.[115]

Gravity will draw the feet into the floor, giving us the anchor that we need to live in the world. For many of us this anchor was missing as our mothers also did not have a connection to their own bodies. As a result, our bodies became misaligned very early on. We learn to compensate in various ways, pulling things out of alignment. Often this unintentionally causes further problems as we grow further away

---

[113] Hymns in the ancient tradition of Indian philosophy dating back approximately to the period between 2500 and 600 B.C.

[114] Rg Veda x, 90, from Sarvepalli Radhakrishnan and Charles A. Moore, eds., *A Sourcebook in Indian Philosophy*, p. 19.

[115] "Problems of Modern Psychotherapy," *The Practice of Psychotherapy*, CW 16, par. 146.

from the central axis designed for us by nature. We can become re-united with the earth, however, and with the Great Mother in all her magnificent glory:

The yearning for the mother can therefore also be understood, in non-mythological language, as the attraction exerted by the unconscious, a constant occurrence that is comparable to the effect of the law of gravity.116

As we continue to breathe roots into the feet, we follow the descent into the underworld of the Sumerian goddess Inanna-Ishtar.[117] Furthermore, in ancient Greece, when there was an unsolved question, people would go down into a cave to hear the prophetic oracle, the idea being that secrets are contained below the surface of the earth.

It is the center of the heels that forms a line with the center of the earth. Breathing into the heels allows the small piece of ground on which one is standing to become firmer and firmer until one begins to feel that one is standing on something really solid. When we reach the center of the earth we cannot go any further down, we have come to "rock bottom," so to speak, we have reached the limit. The more one drops down, the more one feels something stable underneath the feet. The process is unending. One day we come to the joyful moment of realizing that we are actually standing on something solid and that, whatever it is that we have found, cannot be taken away from us. As Jung tells us:

The patient must be alone if he is to find out what it is that supports him when he can no longer support himself. Only this experience can give him an indestructible foundation.118

Standing "rooted" on the earth is truly magnificent. The strength that comes from being rooted is inexpressible in words. Whether standing, sitting or lying down, we feel the immense support of

---

116 Emma Jung and Marie-Louise von Franz, *The Grail Legend*, pp. 42f.
117 See Sylvia Perera, *Descent to the Goddess: A Way of Initiation for Women.*
118 "Introduction to the Religious and Psychological Problems of Alchemy," *Psychology and Alchemy*, CW 12, par. 32.

something holding us from below, which in the end is absolutely irre-
placeable.

Ruth, the forty-year-old woman who had suffered for years from
severe phobic anxieties,[119] had the following dream after three years
of analysis:

> I am in Zurich and I notice that the bone at the back of my foot, in the
> heel, is broken. I call the doctor and he tells me that he can't do anything
> for me. I don't like what he tells me at all as I want to walk into town to
> do some errands. All of a sudden I notice that despite the break in the foot I
> am able to walk. The amazing thing is that I also feel no pain at all.

In the dream Ruth broke her foot right in the area of the tendon
which is named after Achilles, the almost invulnerable Greek hero who
was protected at birth through immersion in holy waters, with the ex-
ception of his heel, the place where he would always remain vulnerable. The heel, in particular the back of the heel where the Achilles
tendon is located, is in reality an extremely delicate part of the foot
that sustains and holds us on the ground. If it is used in the right way,
that is, in tune with gravity, somehow it will protect the body, making
it, if not invulnerable, at least less vulnerable.[120]

During her analysis Ruth learned that her weaknesses are also her
gifts. At the time of this dream she had begun to do things she had
never done before—to go on ski lifts and to ride on trams, carrying
her wounds with her. Ruth began to go out into the world and find the
love for herself that she so desperately longed for.

It is through our vulnerabilities that we remain human. There is a
certain permeability between the divine and the human worlds where
the crossing-over occurs through the medium of the subtle body.
Through our practice both realms become accessible and one bliss-
fully experiences them simultaneously.

---

[119] See above, p. 44.
[120] Scaravelli, *Awakening the Spine*, p. 74.

5
Yaakov

No one should deny the danger of the descent, but it *can* be risked. No one *need* risk it, but it is certain that some will. And let those who go down the sunset way do so with open eyes, for it is a sacrifice which daunts even the gods. Yet every descent is followed by an ascent; the vanishing shapes are shaped anew, and a truth is valid in the end only if it suffers change and bears new witnesses in new images, in new tongues, like a new wine that is put into old bottles.

—C.G. Jung, *Symbols of Transformation.*

It is said in Genesis that after years of longing for a child, Rebekah became pregnant with twins. The twin brothers fought so aggressively while in the womb that Rebekah went to seek the advice of God. It was in a holy place where it is said that God came down to meet his people, thereby uniting divine with human energy. It was here that Rebekah heard the oracle from God:

> Two nations are in thy womb,
> and two peoples shall be separated
>   from thy bowels;
> and the one people shall be stronger than the
>   other people;
> and the elder shall serve the younger.[121]

The prediction that Jacob, the younger brother, would be stronger than Esau, the older, became manifest at their birth:

> And the first came out red, all over like a hairy garment; and they called his name "Esav." And after that came out his brother, and his hand took hold on Esav's heel; and his name was called Ya'aqov.[122]

---

[121] Gen. 25:23.
[122] Gen. 25:25-26.

The name Jacob, *Yaakov* in Hebrew, comes from a word meaning one who takes by the heel or supplants. Etymologically, to supplant means not only to displace but also to bring down, to bring to a low level. This is what is meant by coming down into the heels—that we descend in order to gain strength, which Jacob in fact does.

Another derivation of the word *Yaakov* comes from the root *akov*, meaning crooked. Through our heels we correct the misalignments in our body; we begin to stand in a straight line perpendicular to the earth. When we are properly aligned within the larger energy system around us, we become connected to the positive side of the archetype.

Jacob does in fact supplant his older brother Esau through mercurially deceiving him out of his birthright, thereby receiving the blessing from their father Isaac that was meant for Esau. It is said in the *Mishnah* that after Jacob receives the blessing:

> He, by reason of the blessing he had received, came out crowned like a bridegroom; and the dew which is to revive the dead descended upon him from heaven, his bones became stronger, and he himself was turned into a mighty man.[123]

Through his connection to the heel, Jacob acquires a strong and skillful body like Esau's; he acquires a new status. In the embodiment of the chthonic shadow, Jacob unites the higher spiritual energy with its dark lower counterpart. Jacob embraces life through the transformative, revivifying dew that showers down upon him from heaven. It is as if the bodily vigor that had originally belonged to Esau was taken away and later claimed by Jacob, who was then able to leave the protected world of his past and venture out into the world. The night-sea journey had begun. We must leave our parental complexes behind in order to discover our beloved, within and without. In his impersonation of Esau, Jacob gained a sense of power in his limbs. He had been recreated as had Adam before him; actually the Hebrew word for "bones"—*atzamot*—is closely related to the word for "self."[124] Like

---

[123] *Pirke d'Rabbi Eliezer*, quoted in Heinz Westman, *The Springs of Creativity*, p. 146.

[124] Zornberg, *Genesis: The Beginning of Desire*, p. 178.

Mercurius, Jacob embodies both good and evil; he is shifty and can change his skin at will.

In alchemical Tantric literature a text tells us of the miraculous healing powers of mercury as the divine diamond body: "Thereupon, one becomes [takes on] another body: there is no need to speculate on this matter."[125]

Jacob does in fact change his skin before he goes before his father, thereby cheating his older brother out of the blessing. He gains a thicker, more mature skin which protects him and allows him to enter the world as a man. He experiences a true initiation. Jacob reenacts an age-old ritual where renewal takes place through the imitation of snakes as they cast off their skins. The physical strength and power previously given to Esau is now appropriated by Jacob; the projection is withdrawn.

As diamond-bound mercury is apparently capable of transforming up to ten million times its mass of base metals into gold, it becomes the means of realization of the immortalized body, a body thereby possessed of the power of flight into the beyond, as we see in another alchemical text:

> O Goddess! Swooned, mercury, like the breath, drives away disease; killed, it revives itself; and bound, it affords the power of flight.[126]

Here we come once again to the essential paradox inherent in this work: we must let our bodies release to the Saturn-like heaviness of gravity in order to feel supple and effortless in our corporeal existence. The consequent lightness comes only as we are held by the earth below, otherwise ascending upward in flight may mean surrendering to the dark side of God, ultimately to a profound death wish. This shadow side must be assimilated by taking root in the earth. Paradoxically, we must not lose hold of the wings of Mercurius, remembering that Mercurius, being both "winged" and "wingless,"[127] unites spirit and matter. Again to quote David Gordon White:

---

[125] Quoted in David Gordon White, *The Alchemical Body,* p. 150.

[126] Ibid., p. 149.

[127] See"The Dual Nature of Mercurius," *Alchemical Studies,* CW 13, par. 267.

As we have already seen, the fixing of mercury is also referred to as the clipping of its wings by which it is prevented from volatizing and "flying upwards" (evaporating). Similarly, in yogic practice, it is crucial that the "cosmic goose" of the breaths and vital energy be tethered so as not to leave the body.[128]

Jacob, transformed through the acquisition of a new body "lifted up his feet and went to the land of the people of the east."[129] Unlike Isaac, his father, who waited at home while his future wife was found, Jacob sets out himself on a journey into the vast unknown, truly embodying the masculine principle. Jacob consolidates the blessing by bringing it into reality in the body. Rashi comments on the fact that Jacob lifts up his feet and goes out: "His heart lifted up his legs and he became light on his feet."[130]

Here we see the transformation of the heaviness of Saturn through the medium of dew, the eternal water which brings the gift of the everlasting. It is through the discovery of the body as nature meant it to be, flexible yet ever-present in her beauty, that we connect to the eternity of the soul. In the "Dicta Belini" Dorn quotes Saturn: "My spirit is the water that loosens the rigid limbs of my brothers."[131]

We enter the body through the heart by allowing ourselves to "feel" our way. Paradoxically, when one is truly grounded in the feet through deeply connecting to the heels, lightness and freedom come very naturally into the body. Our feet connect us to what is below. They actually have two primary functions, to support us and to carry us out into the world. The more anchored we are to the ground, and the more secure is the base beneath us, the more we can strive for the light of consciousness. We are told that Jacob's bones become stronger as he attains the "new body," which paradoxically bestows upon him a lightness of foot. In Figure 13 we see what it actually means to hold the opposites in relation to the central axis in the body.

---

[128] *The Alchemical Body*, p. 278.
[129] Gen. 29:1.
[130] Zornberg, *Genesis: The Beginning of Desire*, p. 179.
[131] Quoted in "The Relation of Mercurius to Astrology and the Doctrine of the Archons," *Alchemical Studies*, CW 13, par. 274.

This again brings us back to the notion of *asana* as being firm yet at the same time flexible and relaxed. Paradoxically, simply becoming firm and what we tend to regard as "strong," often involves a rigidity and ensuing stiffness that is not at all what has been originally intended. Vanda Scaravelli expresses this as it manifests in the body:

Practice transforms us . . . . We become more beautiful, our faces change and our walk gains in elasticity. Our way of standing is steady and poised, our legs are firmer, and our toes and feet spread out, giving us more stability. Our chests expand, the muscles of the abdomen start to work, the head is lighter on the neck (like the corolla of a flower on its stem moving easily with flexibility while the wind blows). To watch these enchanting changes is amazing. . . . A different life begins and the body expresses a happiness never felt before. These are not just words, it really happens.[132]

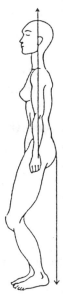

Figure 13. Side view of a woman imagining that her sacrum is so heavy that it actually sinks down toward the ground behind her heels. Simultaneously she is imagining that her central axis is rising upward so that the top of her head moves skyward.

Jacob goes out from the house of his parents in his new skin. He leaves as a bridegroom in search of his bride, able to meet the darkness of the night for the first time. We are told in the Bible that Jacob interrupts his journey for a night's sleep as darkness had fallen upon

---

[132] Quoted by Esther Myers in *Yoga and You*, pp. 26f.

the earth.[133] Here Jacob will encounter the dark night of the soul in the true sense of the word. He will return to the *prima materia* as Adam did when he was plunged into darkness at the close of the first Sabbath. It is said in Torah commentary that the sun had set early that day in order that Jacob might spend the night in the holy place of Luz, which as we saw earlier referred to the eternal "holy bone."[134]

The darkness has come about unexpectedly, intentionally created by God to constellate the *prima materia*, as we read in the Midrash, "to speak to Jacob in private—like a king who calls for the lights to be extinguished, as he wishes to speak to his friend in private."[135]

It is interesting to note that twenty years later, when Jacob returns from exile after struggling with the angel, we are told that the sun rises over him again.[136] According to the same Midrash, this is the first night in fourteen years that Jacob has taken a night's sleep due to his constant preoccupation with the study of the Torah. We are told that Jacob continues to remain awake after this one night of sleep for the duration of the next twenty years that he remains in exile, leaving him in total thirty-four years of sleeplessness, interrupted by this rare night of numinosity. Here Jacob will encounter God through the *experience* of the unconscious (Figure 14).

As Jacob is readying himself to sleep, he gathers the stones around him and places them under his head, preparing for a primordial religious experience. Jacob, as the mercurial mediator between man and God, unites the four elements in divine totality. In the darkness of the night he dreamt:

> And behold a ladder set up on the earth, and the top of it reached to heaven: and behold the angels of God ascending and descending on it.[137]

According to medieval commentary, the ladder was intentionally placed directed toward the earth. It is from the earth that the angels

---

[133] Gen. 28:11.
[134] See above, pp. 71ff.
[135] Quoted in Zornberg, *Genesis: The Beginning of Desire*, p. 187.
[136] Gen. 32:31.
[137] Gen. 28:12.

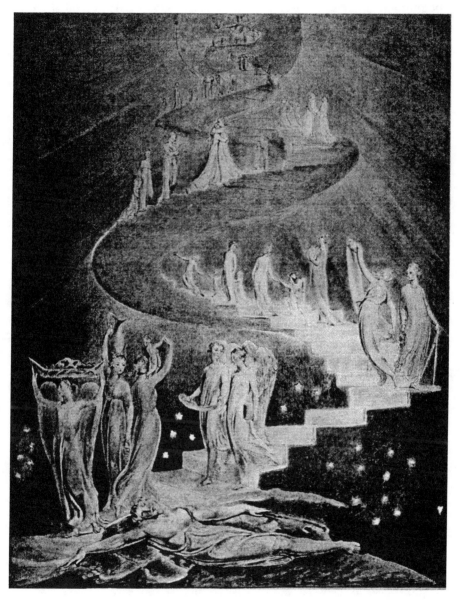

Figure 14. William Blake, "Jacob's Ladder."

begin their up and down movement. Nature herself tells us that it cannot be any other way, it is a natural process that is always present in human beings as well as in all upright living things. The roots of a tree are drawn down deeply toward the center of the earth while the trunk grows upward toward the sky. We take for granted that the deeper the roots impregnate the ground, the taller and stronger the tree is able to grow. The central part of the tree, just at the earth's surface, corresponds to the center of the spine at the level of the fifth lumbar vertebra just above the sacrum, as explained earlier.

We can see in Jung's writings that he did not actually advocate the practice of yoga for his patients as he understood yoga to be *only* a striving upward which he felt, and rightly so, to be dangerous. However, I feel that Jung explains what he means by this warning in a very clear way. We can extrapolate from that explanation that the yoga I am discussing here would not have been considered dangerous in his mind; in fact I believe he would rather have felt it to be the opposite. Grounding and finding the heels in order to bring freedom and suppleness into the upper body can only be extremely helpful, especially in working with people who have never before experienced grounding in their life and who do not live in their bodies. Jung says:

> That canal or shaft she [Christiana Morgan] comes down would be the *sushumna*, the canal through which the Kundalini rises. And here we have the remarkable fact that she is coming down. Here we see the tremendous difference between India and the West. You see, if she tried to go up the *sushumna*, it would be perfectly unnatural, a merely imaginary enterprise. The point is that she is already up above, and what she must establish is below so she must come down. While the East is already below and has to establish a connection with the thing above, because clearness of consciousness does not exist with them, their consciousness is blurred. Therefore the great mistake which Western people make is imitating the Eastern yoga practices, for they serve a need which is not ours; it is the worst mistake for us to try to get higher and higher. What we should do is establish the *connection* between above and below. But we take eagerly to the practice of yoga, which of course does not work; it has very bad effects because our need is just the contrary one. Therefore I always warn people not to

use this Eastern method, for I have never seen a case which was not applied with the wrong purpose of getting still more on top, of acquiring more power or more control, either of their own body, or of other people, or of the world. People use it in order to strengthen their willpower in order to have a hypnotic influence, but that is a dangerous thing to do. The temptation is very great, but happily enough in the majority of cases it has no effect. Our patient is now at the bottom of the well. That would be the *muladhara* in the terminology of the Kundalini yoga system, the root support.[138]

When we are able to drop the heels firmly into the floor, the entire foot finds a place and can rest comfortably and evenly on the ground. We may be inclined to take this statement for granted, but in fact if one looks at feet carefully, one sees that they are rarely evenly sitting on the ground. Photographs of Egyptian statues (Figures 15 and 16)

Figure 15.

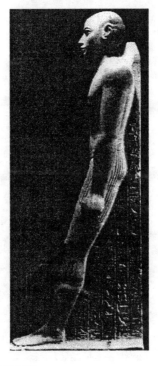

---

[138] *The Visions Seminars*, pp. 598f.

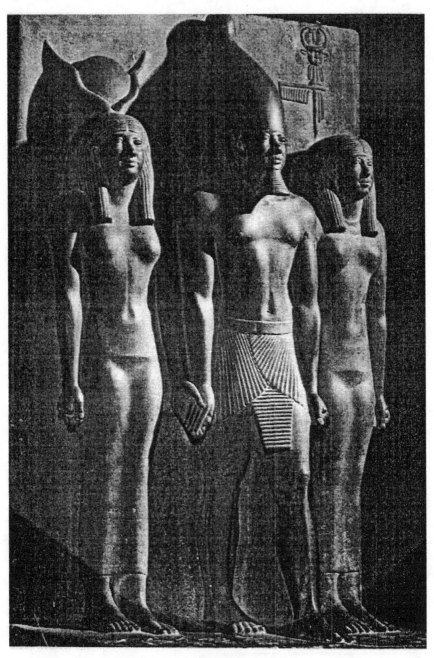

Figure 16.

show the spine as completely straight. There is no curve at the back of the waist. It is at this exact point that the spine divides and moves upward and downward at the same time.

Looking closely at these figures, it can be seen that the Egyptians walked by placing their heels down first while keeping the knees straight, extending the soles of the feet forward from the heels toward the toes. This gave them huge energy, allowing them dignity and poise in their movements. Their power was coming to them from the earth through the soles of the feet which, as centers of vitality and life force, meet and receive energy from the earth.[139]

The divine numinosity that Jacob experienced while in the dream came from his ability to root himself in the heels, which was foreshadowed at his birth. It is through roots in our heels that the ability to travel up and down the spine is produced. Jacob's birth "through the heel," so to speak, foreshadows the strength that will later manifest in his life. We also find our strength through the grounding of the heels, which in turn form the base, the root of the standing yoga postures.

It is imperative that we hold both images of dropping down and rising up simultaneously. Jung reminds us over and over again that it is the *relationship* between the upper and lower worlds that matters, not a straight line that leads to an either-or dilemma which ignores the archetypal world. We know that when spirit incarnates in the world, it must come down to earth. Birth takes place when God descends upon the earth. The light of consciousness always lies above and must always come down to meet matter in the effort to effect a reconciliation of the opposites. Matter itself cannot rise up to meet spirit, it requires the impregnation of spirit in order that it may rise. When we rise up with the wave of the breath, we become infused with spirit as long as we remain in the body, otherwise we lose our connection to the earth and the spirit can no longer be held. It seems that there is too much emphasis on ascension motifs today; we can easily forget, therefore, that we must always remain grounded. The Egyptians represented the theme of ascension by the burial gift of a ladder that would be given

---

[139] Scaravelli, *Awakening the Spine*, pp. 12f.

to the soul of the dead in order to aid entrance into the other world. Rising up signifies the return to god in the heavens. Thus we must remain in the earth, for the earth is our body.

We must never forget our essential connection to gravity, which out of necessity requires the up and down movement in order to elongate, thus gradually entering new areas which would otherwise remain untouched. With his marvellous lucidity, Jung offers us a profound image of what it could really mean to be able to hold both sides at once, thus conquering the one-sidedness of neurosis. As we ground and extend with the wave, as explained earlier,[140] it proves invaluable to keep this image in mind:

> Till Eulenspiegel laughed like mad when he went uphill, and wept when he went downhill. People could not understand it, for wisdom is never understood by ordinary people, but to him it was perfectly clear. In going up he thinks of the descent and that makes him laugh. He rejoices in the idea that soon he will be able to go downhill. But when he goes downhill he foresees that he will soon have to climb again and he weeps therefore.[141]

We are reminded here of the twelfth dream in the series in *Psychology and Alchemy* where the dreamer dreams of a "dangerous walk with Father and Mother, up and down many ladders."[142] Jung suggests that this refers to a process of psychic transformation that necessarily entails many ups and downs. As Father and Mother are specifically mentioned here, it is the personal unconscious that is meant. The contents of the personal unconscious are usually revealed before the contents of the collective unconscious can emerge. Jacob as dreamer embodies the total evolutionary process as an aspect of the Self which incorporates both his personal history as well as that of all mankind. Jacob was chosen to be a messenger of God. A Midrash tells us that Jacob himself is the ladder upon which the angels travel, thereby uniting body and spirit in divine marriage.[143]

---

[140] See above, p. 81.
[141] *Nietzsche's* Zarathustra, p. 226.
[142] "Individual Dream Symbolism in Relation to Alchemy," CW 12, par. 78.
[143] *Bereshit Rabbah*, 68:18, quoted in Zornberg, *Genesis,* p.191.

We could say that Jacob's ego has become strong enough to surrender to the immensity of divine energies, to the Self. He had taken on a new skin, so to speak, which has allowed him to yield to that which was greater within him. The Kabbalists see the ascent both as a process which happens after death and as that which must be preceded by the descent of the soul to Earth in order to be born in the first place. Ascension is the return to the Divine. Each soul is but one tiny cell contained in the body of Adam Kadmon, the Divine Man who comes down into the lower world in order to gain experience. Knowledge and the wisdom gained through experience are imparted to the Divine in the reunion after death. This process continues infinitesimally until Adam Kadmon has become totally aware of all existence. In this way the lower worlds (often represented as the three lower chakras) become a mirror for the divine world above. We as human beings are but a mirror of the divine image.

The aim of Kabbalistic practice is to aid the redemption of both the individual and the collective man as the ultimate manifestation of matter, which in the end is identical to the goal of the alchemists. Meditation was one of the most powerful Kabbalistic practices. As a rule it begins by sitting in stillness on the ground in order to activate energy that is sleeping in *muladhara*, in the first chakra. In the Katha Upanishad 2.21 we are told that sitting in meditation greatly benefits those devoted to the practice:

> Though one sits in meditation in a
> Particular place, the Self within
> Can exercise his influence far away.
> Though still, he moves everything
> everywhere.

6
Muladhara, Elephants and the Kabbalah

The Self brings a feeling of standing on solid ground inside oneself,
on a patch of inner eternity which even physical death cannot touch.
—Marie-Louise von Franz, *C. G. Jung: His Myth in Our Time.*

The path of Kundalini yoga can be a dangerous one, especially for
the Westerner. When one has not received the grounding and security
that are essential in early life, the desire to leave life may be very
strongly constellated. Many people go around half-alive, not knowing
what they want, what they need, or what may be destructive for them.
Embracing life can be so frightening that the split life of ambivalence
is scarcely endured. One fears being caught in earth, in mother, and
never being able to free oneself. Nothing feels more scary to someone
who has never before felt the love of secure arms.

A few years ago a woman in her early forties came to see me concerning a problem, as she told me at that time, of never being in her
body. Louise described her life as almost trancelike and she wanted to
experience what being present in everyday life could mean. She had a
difficult background of early loss and trauma and one could certainly
understand why she had never been able to feel present in the world
around her. Louise came into analysis because she had been unable to
conceive a child for many years and the resultant infertility was put-
ting an almost intolerable stress on her marriage. Furthermore, the
invasiveness of the medical testing echoed the trauma of her past. After about two years of analysis she brought the following dream:

> I was eating a green rat. I could hear the crunching of each little bone as I
> consumed the rat. The green was an iridescent, luminous green.

Together we dwelled on the mystery of this image. Louise had
dreamt about this green rat while on a residential course with a group
of people who were also studying what she loved most in life, the

wonders of nature. She told me that she had felt completely contained by the group and had slept unusually well during this special week.

The rat dream brought Louise back to her archetypal roots, to her origins, to *muladhara*, the base chakra which brings us into the domain of the instincts, into the body. I refer again to Jung:

> When man developed out of that lowest center, *muladhara*, he got into the pre-psychological region, the condition which is characterized by the psychology of emotions.[144]

The color of *muladhara* is a very deep red, the color of passion, of blood, and of life. Marion Woodman suggests that the chakras can be seen in the light of our early existence:

> The chakras may also be interpreted in developmental terms. The root chakra is the survival chakra, a kind of primal hold on life, desiring food, desiring comfort, desiring love—all the basic needs of the young child.[145]

Monica, a woman of sixty-five, had the following dream after a long yoga practice. Her deep early wounding has manifested in terrible shame around her body. She feels that yoga has been a miracle for her and she rarely misses a day of meditation:

> A red setter had joined us. It seemed to have lost its family. I accepted it at first a bit reluctantly but soon found it a very consoling presence. He was a very good dog but also very comforting and reassuring to stroke.

Yoga has given Monica a reason to believe in herself and to believe in a new life opening up to her. It is known in the scientific world that the activation of the life-force takes place in the bloodstream. An electromagnetic current is created by the polarity between the physical and subtle bodies. Somehow there is a connection between the life-force in the blood and the brain which manifests in consciousness but this is not yet understood by modern medicine. In homeopathy, a remedy becomes activated through the life-force that enters the subtle bodies, the chakras, through the various meridians located throughout

---

[144] *The Visions Seminars*, p. 408.
[145] Woodman and Dickson, *Dancing in the Flames*, p. 59.

the body.[146] Through working in *muladhara* we return to our beginnings. It is as if, paradoxically, while being securely grounded in the
earth, we are being transported back in time.

Muladhara is the foundation, the building block upon which all
other chakras must rest. In *muladhara* a lotus flower is represented
with four petals, within which a circle has been squared, representing
the fifth element, the *quinta essentia* that creates the immortal body
through the transformative *luz* bone (Figure 17).

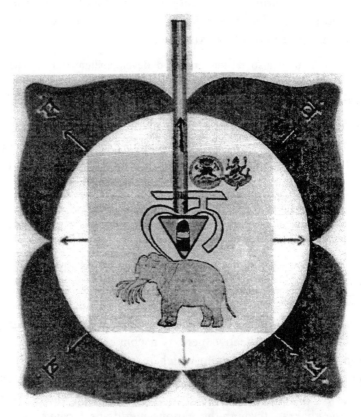

Figure 17. The *muladhara* chakra.

---

[146] A meridian is a channel carrying subtle energy *(ch'i)* to the body's various organs, nerves and blood vessels.

The ability to turn a square into a circle was one of the preoccupations of the alchemists, in other words, to reach a union of opposites by bringing heaven and earth together into one entity. Squaring the circle or circling the square, whichever way we want to think of it, is the embodiment of the circular aspect of the heavens that is transforming into the earth, and vice versa.

The process of spiraling up and down is a never-ending one. The squaring of a circle represents an irrational state of wholeness which, in order to be integrated, must be experienced in the subtle body. In "The Visions of Zosimos," Jung tells us that Dorn maintained that the squaring of a circle produced the sacred alchemical vessel, in which all and everything takes place.[147] Dorn goes on to say that the creation of the vessel is essentially a psychic operation; it is the creation of an inner readiness that will accept the Self as standing behind the whole process. Here the vessel is beautifully contained in the fifth element within the four-petaled lotus structure. The number four reminds us of the dust that God gathered from the four corners of the world in order to make the primordial man, Adam Kadmon. The material world is based on the wholeness inherent in the earth. The four petals can also be seen as representing the four elements of the material kingdom: earth, water, fire and air.

Within the square in Figure 17 is a small triangle pointing downward from a column of energy representing the *susumna*,[148] symbolizing the downward energy force contained in this chakra. If one looks carefully, one can see that within this triangle there lies the Kundalini serpent wrapped around the *lingam* (phallus) of Shiva which points upward toward consciousness. Above and below are magnificently united. Below the triangle sits the magnificent *Airavata*, the seven-trunked elephant who represents the instinctual quality in the body that is prevalent in this chakra. One finds that often the elephant-headed god, Ganesha, is associated with *muladhara*.

---

[147] *Alchemical Studies*, CW 13, par. 115.
[148] *Susumna* is the central channel in Kundalini yoga that connects the chakras to each other; it is also called the "royal road" to enlightenment.

Looking back at Louise's dream where she is eating a green rat, we note that Ganesha, the Indian elephant god of obstacles, was often depicted as sitting above a rat. It is common in Indian iconography to find an animal symbol placed beneath an anthropomorphic god. Here the rat, who carries the elephant, so to speak, is called the "vehicle." The rat can thus be seen as the personality and energy of the god Ganesha. One can imagine the strength of character that the rat must have in order to be able to carry the entire weight of the elephant on its back. The rat, like his divine counterpart Ganesha, is also said to be able to overcome obstacles and is therefore a fitting animal to carry the god. The elephant passes through the wilderness, treading on shrubs, bending and uprooting trees, easily fording rivers; the rat can gain access to the bolted granary. The two together represent the power of this god to overcome every obstacle in its way.[149] One can surmount almost any impediment when survival is not threatened, when contained in *muladhara*.

For Louise, eating the green rat meant the beginning of an integration of the elements of *muladhara* that had been so lacking in her life. Her body has become strong and more able to meet what was previously very difficult for her. In other words, her instinctual life was becoming available to her, bringing her into relationship with her body and with her feminine nature.

The elephant proves to be a complicated animal because it is so big. As it is far heavier than any other animal on land, it not only needs pillars for legs but literally an acre of lung surface to absorb oxygen, an eight-foot trunk to reach its food, a massive heart to circulate blood, and hundreds of feet of guts and complex digestive organs to assimilate nourishment from the hundreds of pounds of foliage and grass it eats every day.

Since time immemorial, the elephant has walked the earth. According to ancient Indian cosmology, eight celestial elephants protected the eight points of the compass in the sky. Their descendants had wings and, like clouds, they roamed freely in the skies. This idyl-

---

[149] See Heinrich Zimmer, *Myths and Symbols in Indian Art and Civilization*, p. 70.

lic condition could not remain forever; many lost their wings through carelessness. Ever since that time, the elephant has been forced to remain on the ground.[150] These huge animals archetypally represent both winged and wingless creatures, thus carrying the attributes of both; they can fly in the air and produce clouds which later fill with rain and thus release the gifts from the unconscious upon the earth. Elephants can be thought of as rain-clouds walking upon the earth, making them suitable bridges between heaven and the earth.

Muladhara, literally meaning "root support," provides an ideal seat for the elephant to serve as the divine carrying power within the first chakra. In a classic eighth-century monument of Hindu religious architecture, The Temple of the Lord of Mount Kailasa, the elephant is used as the supporting column itself (Figure 18). The whiteness of *Airavata*, the elephant which sits at the base of the square within *muladhara*, suggests that the origin of this "milk" elephant is the result

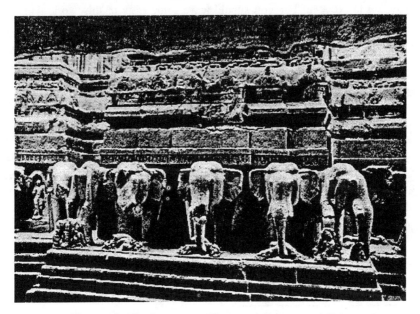

Figure 18. Elephant caryatids (seventh century A.D.)

---

[150] Ibid., p. 106.

of the churning of the milk in the Hindu creation myth that eventually produces *amrita*, the potion that guarantees immortality. Before the agitation of the milk could begin, a churning pole was necessary; it was deemed good by the gods and demons of that time to use the mountain *Mandara* expressly for that purpose. *Mandara* was 77,000 miles high, with roots that went an equal distance into the earth. *Mandara* is the spine that extends infinitely in two opposing directions, giving us but a tiny glimpse of the eternal world to come.

Being in *muladhara* means coming into a relationship with reality and connecting to the roots of our existence. When we practice yoga we ourselves become the roots that deeply penetrate into the earth. As Jung explicitly tells us:

> You must believe in this world, make roots, do the best you can. . . . but you have to believe in it, have to make it almost a religious conviction, merely for the purpose of putting your signature under the treaty, so that a trace is left of you. For you should leave some trace in this world which notifies that you have been here, that something has happened. If nothing happens of this kind you have not realized yourself; the germ of life has fallen, say, into a thick layer of air that kept it suspended. It never touched the ground, and so never could produce the plant. But if you touch the reality in which you live, and stay for several decades, if you leave your trace, then the impersonal processes can begin.[151]

As we become the roots that descend into the earth, we come into contact with the feminine, with the body, which is referred to in the Kabbalah as the *Shekhinah*, the incarnated divine feminine presence on earth. She is the principal feminine aspect manifesting within herself the source of all life. As the *Shekhinah* is embodied, she is capable of being perceived. She is the mother who repeatedly intercedes on behalf of her children. She is *Malkhut*, who dwells at the bottom of the Sefirotic Tree (Figure 19),[152] gathers all of the emanations from the world above, and serves as the mirror and container in which all

---

[151] *The Psychology of Kundalini Yoga*, p. 29.

[152] The *sefiroth* are the ten essences of energy in Kabbalistic thought that bring the world into being through the unfolding of the essence of God. On the Tree of Life they represent the lights of the attributes of God.

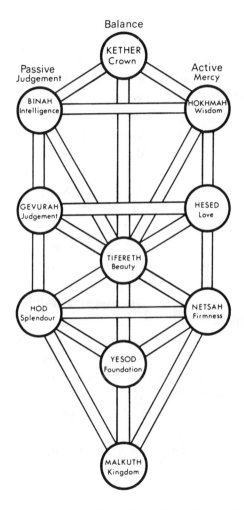

Figure 19. The Sefirot, Kabbalistic Tree of Life.

lights issuing from this emanative structure are absorbed.[153]

> The ten Sefirot appear out of Nothing like a Lightning Flash or scintillating flame, and they are without beginning or end. The Name of God is with them as they go forth and when they return.[154]

Malkhut is known as the "daughter" or the "Kingdom," the place where the body exists in the reality of the material world. It is said that when the *Shekhinah* is present the silence of the spiritual dimension is broken, giving way to divine speech. It is the voice that makes the body come alive.

All of the higher sefirot flow into *Malkhut* where the *Shekhinah* waits to be united with her bridegroom, for she is an abandoned widow, so to speak,[155] and therefore incomplete without him. She is the awaited partner of Jacob who, akin to Mercurius, is the bridegroom wrapped up in the eternal search for his bride.

As we come into contact with the lowest chakra we are confronted with the primal fear of abandonment, with being a widow, facing the bleakness of being truly alone. This is only an illusion, however, as we are all essentially alone; so we are born and so we die. It is only through being connected to the archetypal world that we are able to feel a loving container around us. Gradually, as we continue to work in *muladhara*, within the divine presence of the *Shekhinah*, we learn to stand alone in the face of our greatest difficulties. When we are truly able to meet the feminine aspect within, we begin to develop a relationship to the world around us. To be in the world is to have an ego and to know that the ego has only been given to us as an instrument for the revelation of divine energy, not as an end in itself. We can gradually allow ourselves our vulnerabilities while remaining strongly contained within *muladhara*.

---

[153] Emanation in Kabbalistic thought is the coming into being of the universe through the unfolding of God's essence in a series of ten stages, the spheres of *sefirot*.

[154] From the *Sefer Yezirah* (an early work of Jewish mysticism), quoted in Z'ev ben Shimon Halevi, *Adam and the Kabbalistic Tree*, p. 25.

[155] See "The Components of the Coniunctio," *Mysterium Coniunctionis*, CW 14, par. 18.

When *Malkut* is united with her masculine counterpart, it is said that she becomes the "statue," animated through his divine breath of life.[156] The body comes to life. Survival then becomes something we can take for granted. It is solely the breath, or prana, that enlivens us. Only the breath can bring transformation; all other attempts to change the body are of no avail as the gift of life is absent. Breath is the manifestation of the life force and sustains us in the eternal realm, as it says in the Kaushitaki Upanishad, III.2:

> Life is prana, prana is life. So long as prana remains in this body, so long is there life. Through prana, one obtains, even in this world, immortality.[157]

The way we breathe, whether it be shallow or deep, slow or fast, depends not only on actual training but on our psychological conditions, as Jung proved over and over again in his use of the association experiment. With each breath we create new life; something new is born each time that we take a breath.

In the sixteenth century, when Jewish mysticism was flourishing in Palestine, Isaac Luria introduced a radically different vision of the Creation myth and of the place of the individual within it. He imagined that before God created the world He actually drew himself in, or contracted, in order to leave space for the world in which human beings could live. Within that space were tiny vessels filled with numinous sparks of divine light which were said to contain the future souls of mankind. The energy in the light was too intense, however, shattering the vessels and scattering the sparks in all directions throughout the universe. It is our task to immerse ourselves in the redemptive task of gathering up the sparks of light, thus assisting the divine work of making the universe whole again. It is the universal aim of yoga to attain this new dimension of consciousness which in establishing the birth of a new personality will be compatible with both the tangible and mystical worlds.

It must be emphasized again that it is *not* the goal of yoga to escape

---

[156] See above, p. 57.

[157] Quoted in Georg Feuerstein, *Yoga: The Technology of Ecstasy*, p. 127.

from the material world but rather to bring the worlds of spirit and matter together. As Rabbi Abraham Joshua Heschel reminds us:

> The body is the discipline, the pattern, the law;
> the spirit is inner devotion, spontaneity, freedom.
> A body without a spirit is a corpse
> and a spirit without a body is a ghost.[158]

When we breathe consciously, we create a vacuum in which light can enter at the end of each exhalation. Within this void is contained our whole potential for the development of consciousness. With each breath we reenact the creation of the world. Light enters the darkness of matter. As we continue to breathe while constantly focusing on an inner awareness, the light constellated within will cause the spine to lengthen and grow into itself. Figure 20 represents what the inside of

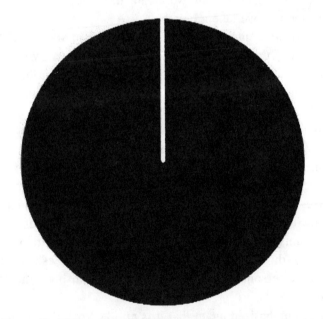

Figure 20. The ray of light of infinity entering the vacated space
of the *Tzimtzum* (contraction).

---

[158] *God in Search of Man: A Philosophy of Judaism*, p. 341.

the belly, the *hara*, would look like at the end of the exhalation when the breath has completely left the body and we are waiting for the new breath to come in, always in its own time.

Actually, Figure 20 is a Kabbalistic image of the Creator in a state of contraction in order to leave space for the creation of the world. By imitating this act over and over again, we create positive energy through releasing toxins and cleansing the body of its impurities. From this single ray of light that enters the body, the ten concentric circles of the Sefirotic Tree evolve and spiral out, filling the world with light, light which has first been grounded in *muladhara*. The ten "lit" sefirot correspond to the ten times that God spoke in the first chapter of Genesis: "Let there be light," through which the world was created and continues to be created with each breath. It is our work to consciously gather the light that was lost when these vessels shattered. We must remember that what has been broken can be healed and that it is necessary to break things apart so that they may come together again. In terms of the body, alignment must be corrected so that we can return to our original posture in the structure of the primordial man, back to nature, to how our bodies were created to be. This is what in the Kabbalah is termed *tikkun*, which refers to the restoration of the disjointed state of humankind to its former harmony and unity.

In order for something to come into being, God must retreat inside himself. When an empty space has been created for the new energy to enter, beams of light are directed into the vacuum, thereby building the world. Breathing in this conscious, concentrated way brings us back over and over again to the nothingness that becomes light that permeates everywhere. This light, however, must be contained within the strong yet flexible vessel that allows for the containment of spirit. When light is sought after purely for its own sake, psychic danger may result.

It is said that the breaking of the vessels is the primordial catastrophe, and that the subsequent restoration of cosmic order is the rectification or redemption of the newly created world. After these vessels that had acquired too much light had shattered, the main stream of light reascended to its origin in the heavens and the light remaining descended into the world where we now live. It is our task to restore this fragmented world to harmony, to bring the wholeness from the world above down into our world, thereby creating a miraculous alignment between heaven and earth. It is in this way that we bring the divine in its mystical holiness into our lives. Holiness must be experienced in apparently insignificant daily tasks in order to have meaning. We must remember that God is always in search of humanity in order to bring about the union of the temporal and the sacred. It is as if God were unwilling to be alone, that His work would be incomplete without us. The search for God is not only our concern but also God's. It is not exclusively a human yearning.

When Adam and Eve hid from God after they had partaken of the forbidden fruit, God called out to them: "Where art thou?"[159]

This call can be heard over and over again in the Bible, not always in words, but repeatedly conveyed to us in mysterious ways. Indeed, we are continually hearing God's question and being challenged to find our own answers.

As we continue to follow the breathing, the point at the end of the exhalation deepens as the abdominal muscle extends back as far as it can go with each breath. It is essential to remember that the exhalation is our primary concern, as it is our precious instrument for the release and letting go of tension. And with this letting go may come feelings that have been repressed in the body for years. The deeper the exhalation is able to go, the more passive will be the following inhalation. Coming into tune with this regular rhythmic breathing allows us to gradually come into our natural way of being, to feel the gift of being truly alive. When the breath is disciplined, we are refusing to breathe just like the majority of mankind; we depart from the collective way and find our unique essence within.

As we continue, the end of the exhalation begins to feel as if the abdomen were being sucked back, as if gravity becomes stronger with each exhalation, pulling one deeper and deeper into the center of gravity, into *muladhara*. With each breath we gather the light into our-

---

[159] Gen. 3:9.

selves, into our roots, thus facilitating our own personal redemption as well as the redemption of the world. Change itself always begins with the individual and it is only through the effort of each one of us that changes in collective consciousness can be brought about.

Rootlessness is widespread in our culture today. It seems as if we are all dependent on something or someone else for our survival. Being grounded in *muladhara*, however, involves the ability to stand on our own two feet, knowing that whatever comes to us in life will be supported not only by ourselves alone, but also by something which is bigger than we can ever be. Being in *muladhara* also involves being in contact with the *prima materia*, that mysterious essence which constellates the life force. All our work ultimately begins and ends in *muladhara*, in the *prima materia*. According to the thirteenth-century Jewish mystic, Rabbi David ben Yehuda, man was created out of clay by the potter who dwells in *Malkuth*, the lowest chakra. Here the *materia* has innumerable possibilities of shape and form. We have not yet become who God has meant us to be. As it is said:

> She [*Knesset Yisrael*—the collectivity of Israel, a feminine entity sometimes equated with the *Shekhinah*] is called the Potter; just as a potter who shapes and fashions clay vessels, making them narrow or wide on the potter's wheel, as it is written: *Like clay in the hand of the potter* [so are you in My hand, O House of Israel] (Jeremiah 18:6).[160]

As we empty the breath at the end of each exhalation, we perceive the void within the vessel of the five-flowered sacrum. We pause, and we inhale the light into the containing vessel of our own reality. As we are filled with golden light the transcendent enters the sacral area and begins to pervade our whole being. In *Malkuth*, or *muladhara* as we are calling it here, the divine essence becomes realized through the personification of the *Shekhinah* as clay vessel, thereby embodying the creative, the *prima materia*. Light must be embodied to engender creation.

---

[160] David ben Yehuda ha-Hasid, *The Book of Mirrors*, quoted in Freema Gottlieb, *The Lamp of God*, p. 299.

Nowadays many spiritual disciplines encourage their aspirants to get away from life, perhaps to retire to a quiet place and meditate. In the tradition of Jewish mysticism, however, the student is advised to live in the midst of the world, in the reality of life. We remember the advice of the ancient sages who have come before and who always urged us to eat bread with salt (which symbolizes the bitterness that must be encountered in the mundane world), to drink water moderately, to sleep on the ground, to lead a close life (meaning a life of reflection), and to study hard.[161] In fact, one is not allowed to embark on the study of Kabbalah without first having a grounding in life, a grounding in reality which, it is said, cannot happen before the age of forty. In fact the sages warned that only the most stable aspirants should undertake the path of Kabbalah.

The same holds true for the pursuit of Kundalini yoga. The dangers of such a path are enumerated throughout yogic texts. A relation to the body must be maintained at all times. Missing the link with the physical level is both uncomfortable and potentially dangerous. The ego must be strong enough to surrender to a higher power. It is with the awakening of the Kundalini serpent that the ego becomes aware that there is something larger than itself. It becomes aware of the Self.

---

[161] See Perle Epstein, *Kabbala: The Way of the Jewish Mystic*, p. xvii.

7
The Fire of Kundalini

As far as we can discern, the sole purpose of human existence
is to kindle a light in the darkness of mere being.
—C. G. Jung, *Memories, Dreams, Reflections.*

An ancient yoga text tells us of the Kundalini serpent as she lies
sleeping at the base of the spine:

> Now there is a compound bone which forms a four-finger wide platform
> [for the spinal column]. It is located two-fingers above the anus and one
> finger below the genitals. Upon this platform, placed in the rear of the
> pelvic region, is to be found the *Kundalini,* coiled three and a half times
> around the root of the *nadis,* lying like a serpent with its tail in its mouth,
> and blocking the entrance of the *Susumna nadi.*
>
> Here she lies asleep, glowing with her own light; and guarding the cru-
> cial junction [of sacrum and the tail end of the backbone] where lies the
> Seed of Speech.[162]

Various methods for the awakening of Kundalini have been described for thousands of years. Although it is generally thought that
she sleeps in *muladhara,* in Jung's view the Kundalini serpent is located in the lumbar area just above the sacrum.[163] I am inclined to
agree with Jung, as that places the Kundalini energy directly at that
crucial point of the fifth lumbar vertebra, the *quinta essentia,* where a
tremendous amount of energy sits, awaiting the birth of consciousness. Widespread opinion has it, however, that the Kundalini serpent
sleeps in *muladhara,* which positions it directly in the center of the
chthonic world, in the fecundity of the earth.

When Kundalini awakens, she hisses and straightens herself into an
upright position, constellating an intense heat that is said to burn as it

---

[162] Siva-Samhita, verses 80-82, quoted in Schyam Gosh, *The Original Yoga,* p. 86.
[163] *The Visions Seminars,* p. 276.

travels up the spine. We can feel this heat ourselves, not only within Kundalini, but in any type of bodywork where, after working for a time at a deep cellular level, we can feel the heat in our body which indicates that a profound change is taking place. Nothing can transform without the alchemical fire. When we live in the fire of our emotions, in the fire of life, something moves through us. Perhaps it is something old that needs to be eliminated, perhaps something new and unfamiliar is thrusting its way in with a blaze of passionate energy. In the East it is said that when one is in communication with God, one burns with love of the divine.

We are told that the serpent lies dormant, coiled three-and-a-half times around and blocking the entrance to the opening of the *susumna* nadi.[164] With the awakening of the Kundalini, the spine straightens as the instinctual world is constellated.

At first glance, this whole process seems simple enough. But we must not take the process of emerging consciousness lightly. Above all, consciousness entails a huge responsibility. Going back to the Axiom of Maria—"One becomes two, two becomes three, and out of the third comes the one as the fourth"—we recall that four is also the one, the number of wholeness, of conscious totality. As four symbolizes the fulfillment of the realization of consciousness and the goal of the work, there is always a hesitation, or what I might rather call an ambivalence, involved in the transition from three to four. As the unconscious is invariably striving for wholeness, however, there is always an inclination toward moving to the four. Remembering that the ultimate aim of analysis is to become conscious, we find that over and over again on our way we experience suffering that must be met each time with boundless faith and courage. It is natural to experience some hesitation on the journey. This is what I believe is meant by the hesitation between the third and the fourth, although in the end, I repeat, there is always an inclination toward the four, toward conscious

---

[164] The nadis are the channels of energy in the subtle body that conduct the prana energy. There are three major nadis: *ida, pingala* and the *susumna* nadi which serves as the central connecting channel to the entire chakra system.

totality. It may sometimes feel tempting just to sit back and let life take over, so to speak, rather than face the problems that coming to consciousness will bring.

This is the ambivalence between the third and the fourth that the Kundalini serpent embodies. She lies coiled three and a half times around the *susumna* nadi, unsure as to whether to begin her ascent toward consciousness. The Kundalini serpent symbolizes, therefore, an aspiration toward wholeness that hesitates and holds back just long enough until the precise moment when the time is right to begin movement. The psyche always has its own timing.

We remember that typologically there is always a deficiency in consciousness if the fourth function is left out. Three is characterized by an unconsciousness of the inferior function. This is seen in the rejection of the body by the Judeo-Christian tradition. The inferior function is the least conscious function and, therefore, not clearly at the disposal of the conscious mind. For that reason the inferior function cannot depend on the ego alone, it is inherently connected to the Self. As it can never become completely conscious, the inferior function always seems to lag behind the other three. This statement is crucial to the understanding of bodywork. As the body is inferior for most of us, especially those of us who are intuitives, we can now see clearly that, as the body is in fact slower than the psyche to transform, it must be treated accordingly. It is often necessary, therefore, that we give more attention to the body than to psyche, if only until the body has a chance to catch up.

If we are truly *in* our body, we can often feel the pull to remain unconscious and at the same time we feel the tremendous urge that propels us forward toward consciousness. In this dormant state, the three and the four remain in conflict until the life force emerges that is able to move the situation to a new level. The serpent always represents a new danger as she embodies our past histories, both in a personal and in a collective way. The most dangerous point, however, is when the serpent reaches the crown of the head in her ascent where there exists the very real danger of flying up into spirit and abandoning the body altogether. It is primarily for this reason that I advocate only the type of yoga that I discuss here or a similar one where the connection with the ground remains first and foremost. Then we will be able to stay in the body while at the same time embracing the numinosity of the spirit, allowing, as Jung says many times over, a complete renewal of the personality.

The fluctuation between the three and four activates the energy that moves continuously back and forth between the spiritual and physical realms, three being the number of the masculine and of the Holy Spirit, and four being the number of the feminine. Serpents are associated with the feminine, resulting from their earthbound, rhythmically undulating movements, as well as from their ability to shed their skin periodically which connects them with the cyclic changes of the moon. In shedding its skin, the serpent manifests the potential for transformation through the continuous cycle of birth, death and rebirth. In choosing the path of consciousness, the Kundalini serpent seems in an uncanny way to possess a mystical knowledge that remains all but incomprehensible to our human understanding. When we recall the fall from Paradise in the Garden of Eden, we see that the serpent is the power behind the development of consciousness. Ultimately the Kundalini serpent is *in potentia* as she sleeps, awaiting the call from the divine. The Kundalini serpent is *embodied* spirituality.

Another text says that when the serpent sleeps, "as if stupefied by a poison," the Kundalini becomes identified with human mortality and the bondage of the ignorant.[165] Subjectively speaking, one becomes paralyzed, the fertilizing creative semen is sucked away, and Medusa has hold. Being under the influence of the poison from the negative mother, there is an ever-present temptation to remain childish and neglect the growth demanded by consciousness. As Sibylle Birkhäuser-Oeri notes, poison is the weapon that is mostly used by women whereas men usually attack their enemies openly. The effects of poison are invisible and insidious.[166] When the body is unconscious, it

---

[165] Lilian Silburn, *Kundalini: Energy of the Depths*, quoted in David Gordon White, *The Alchemical Body*, p. 219.
[166] *The Mother: Archetypal Image in Fairy Tales*, p. 37.

also may remain under the influence of poisonous substances that will bring about illness if the toxins do not find a means of release from the body. Connecting to the Kundalini energy within aligns us to the positive mother who nurtures and gives life, and who simply rejoices in the sheer joy of being alive. An Indian legend tells of Matsyendranath, a hero who had his life force drained away as punishment for years of debauchery and who was fated to die within three days if his consort could not rouse him, in other words, awaken his Kundalini.[167]

The serpent was sacred to Asclepius, the Greek god of medicine. His connection to the serpent is once again primarily associated with the feminine and his counsel was much sought after by childless women. Women would flock to his sanctuary in a beautiful valley to seek his help. As Jacob did, the women would go to sleep in a holy place and in their dreams they would be visited by a serpent who was presumed to be the god himself. The children that were subsequently born to these women were considered to be the offspring of Asclepius himself. Apparently he had assumed the form of a serpent in order to be closer to earth and more accessible to the diseases he treated.[168] In the Eleusinian Mysteries, initiates had to kiss a snake, symbolizing their union with the chthonic principle.[169]

The Kundalini serpent evokes the chthonic aspect of matter where she meets spirit, as bride meets bridegroom. In Egyptian mythology a serpent was considered valuable if it had its head upright, whereas evil serpents crawled flat on the earth. It is the unique ability of the Kundalini serpent to act as a vehicle of transformation through the sudden increase of heat and light that penetrates the darkness of matter. As the Kundalini lies in waiting, the god and goddess, Shiva and Shakti, lie dormant, entwined in a blissful symbiotic state, trapped in the unconsciousness of matter. They are without experience; they have not yet lived. As mentioned earlier,[170] gods have never had the experience

---

[167] White, *The Alchemical Body*, p. 219.
[168] M. Oldfield Howey, *The Encircled Serpent*, pp. 92f.
[169] Gotthilf Isler, *"The Kiss of the Snake,"* p. 13.
[170] See above, p. 42.

of reality as they have no body. It is only through lived experience of being *in* the body that freedom may be gained from enslavement to our complexes.

Christiana Morgan, whose visions and paintings formed the basis of Jung's *Vision Seminars,* painted a vision of a man and woman lying together in a womblike state, enclosed by a circular image of a snake (Figure 21). Here the masculine and feminine are enclosed in a pre-conscious state that resembles the condition of Shiva and Shakti before Shiva has initiated the birth of consciousness. This is the condition of the *prima materia* at the beginning where all the possibilities and mysteries of life have yet to be discovered. The couple are encircled by the snake that lies at the base of the spine, awaiting entrance into life.

Turning to an image of another of Jung's patients (Figure 22), we can see here that the number four has been constellated in the inner circle which has been divided into four parts, thus providing the initiative for the serpent to try to get out of its condition and move into new territories. Jung notes that the arrows outside the circle are pointing outward, which shows the direction in which the snake is trying to go. These two pictures give us clear images of the dormant condition of the Kundalini serpent and its resulting attempt to leave its unconscious state and aspire toward wholeness.

In order to activate the latent energy in the Kundalini, I believe two things must happen. Initially, Shiva must kindle the fire that starts the whole process going and propels the Kundalini to leap up and begin moving. Kundalini is aroused particularly by a spark of fire that constellates in *muladhara*, the instinctual realm. It is the fire that brings spirit to matter, the fire of light within the dark recesses of the root chakra. The life force becomes activated through the intake of breath, the spark of life that brings consciousness to instinctual life. The redness becomes a brilliant burning red that sends sparks urging the Kundalini on to the crown chakra, *quinta essentia* of spirit.

Secondly, enough energy must accumulate in this *muladhara*-lumbar area to awaken the serpent. This happens through a "damming up" of the energy, as is mentioned in *The Secret Of The Golden*

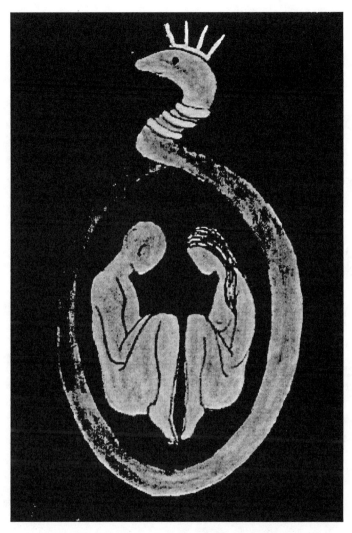

Figure 21. "A man and a woman lying as if in a womb
and about them was coiled a snake."

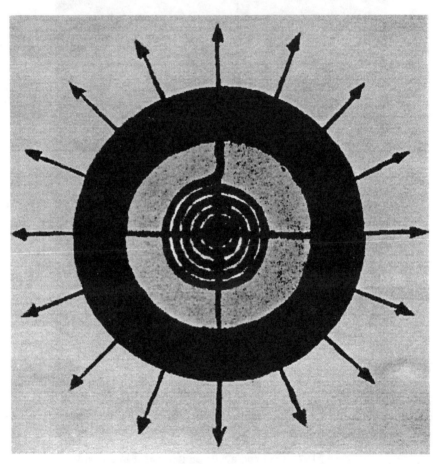

Figure 22.

Flower.[171] When something comes in to stop the natural flow of energy in the body, the energy accumulates until the opposite pole is constellated causing a reversal of the flow of energy toward its source. This is what ultimately happens with the Kundalini such that when enough energy has been stored, the serpent energy begins to rise of its own accord.

The question remains: how do we gather this energy together? The hatha yoga texts prescribed a combination of postures *(asanas)* as well as specific breathing techniques, all aimed at the immobilization and retention of the breath that would then trigger the rise of the Kundalini. It is not possible to discuss all the methods here but we can say that when we have a conscious relationship with the breath, then something can happen. What we are doing is also bringing the focus of awareness inward, allowing all and everything to be gathered and worked on within the alchemical vessel of our body.

Specifically, the inhalation always remains passive, thus receiving the energy impregnated with prana, the external manifestation of the life force. Each time that we exhale down into the sacral area, part of the breath is stored, accumulating energy to prepare for the next breath. In this way the breath deepens, reaching down to the innermost cellular level where transformation can take place at the archetypal level. When the direction of the energy flow reverses, opposing sources of energy are constelled. The goal will be to eventually unite these pairs of opposites, the downward heavier energy and the lighter more upward one. The downward, backward-flowing energy connects us to matter and the upward, lighter energy to spirit. Spirit and matter may once again unite in glorious harmony.

One of the basic yoga *asanas* is the tree pose which involves standing on one leg with all the weight being placed on the standing foot. It is a very important posture for us because as one of the standing balancing poses, it helps us regain our center and teaches us a feeling of being supported by our legs and feet. It is not easy to balance all the weight on one leg and then on the other (when doing the

---

[171] Richard Wilhelm, trans. *The Secret of the Golden Flower,* p. 15, note 1.

reverse side), so that when one eventually comes back to standing in *tadasana,* a sense of aliveness in the legs brings a great feeling of inner stability. In becoming a tree, ideally one comes to rest, remaining utterly quiet within. As soon as movement ceases, the opposites come into balance with one another, bringing harmony within. Christiana Morgan described such a vision to Jung (Figure 23).[172]

In her vision, she has become a tree. Her feet have become the roots, her body the trunk, and her arms the branches that reach upward toward the sun. Her journey toward consciousness had begun. She had incorporated the image of the tree into her body.

Louise, the woman who dreamt that she was eating a green rat,[173] had a similar vision one day in a bodywork session that we did together. After doing a visualization exercise that involved trying to bring light into her body, she found that the light would not travel through her right leg from the knee down. At that moment I asked her to put a positive image into the blocked place,[174] and a tree suddenly appeared and began to push the leg way beyond its normal length. She felt as if an entire tree was growing inside her right leg that suddenly began to develop its own shape and form and to take on a life of its own. After this extraordinary experience, Louise found that her creative energy was on fire in an entirely new way. She tells me that often when she is lying breathing on the floor the tree comes in spontaneously, bringing new creative energy.

The tree is the *quinta essentia* of the union of opposites, of the upper and lower realms, of spirit and matter. The tree embodies the opposites of heaven and earth. Trees receive their nourishment from both above and below, from sunlight and from the water in the earth. The point where Louise was able to become a tree demonstrates that she was coming into her own essence. After all, no tree is like any other; they are all symbols of individual uniqueness.

---

[172] *The Visions Seminars*, p. 248.
[173] See above, pp. 102f.
[174] This follows the work developed by Woodman, Skinner and Hamilton in bodysoul rhythms, as mentioned above in chap. 3.

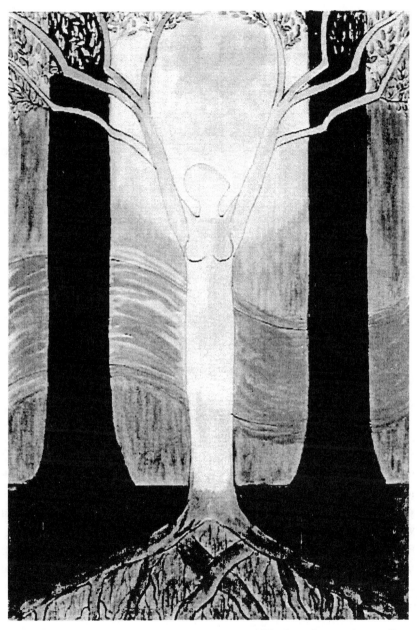

Figure 23. "I knew I had become a tree and lifted my face to the sun."

There are many legends concerning human beings that are born from trees. Trees also connect us to death; we will end our life inside a tree if we choose to be buried in a coffin. Trees have a marvellous dual nature. Being feminine, they can give birth but they can also be phallic as is shown in the alchemical portrait of Adam with the tree growing out of his body as a phallus (Figure 24).

The tree roots us strongly to earth and connects us to *muladhara*, to our ability to survive on our own. What plants and trees really have to teach us is autonomy, for they are the only living things that can exist completely by themselves. When we become a tree, we come into a quiet place of trust, of knowing who we are now and who we may become. Silence is the cherished secret of all the yoga poses. When we remain absolutely still we experience the exquisiteness of the breath as transformer of the subtle body as the Kundalini is activated. The wakening of the Kundalini is not simply the arousal of a dormant force within us, as Gopi Krishna explains:

> The arousal of kundalini, in its true sense, does not simply imply the activity of a hitherto sleeping force, but actually the start of a new activity by changing the whole system to adapt it to a new pattern of consciousness through changing the composition of the bioenergy or subtle life force permeating the whole body.[175]

When we become a tree, we surrender to a fundamental law governing the growth of all plants, that they all grow in spiral formations. The spiral pulls us in two directions at once, back into the womb of our past and simultaneously pushing ahead, yearning for reunion with the divine. Each complete breath we take turns in on itself constantly expanding and contracting as we inhale, as we exhale. Everything that expands must contract, and vice versa. The Sanskrit word *Kundalini* means literally "of a spiral nature," directly implying a double spiral that moves up and down in constant motion. Etymologically, the long *i* added to the Sanskrit adjective *kundalin*, meaning "circular, spiral, coiling, winding," makes a feminine noun signifying "snake," the

---

[175] *Living With Kundalini: The Autobiography of Gopi Krishna*, p. 35.

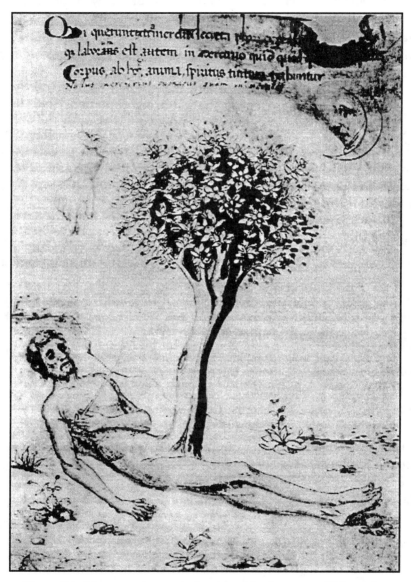

Figure 24. Adam as *prima materia*, pierced by the arrow of Mercurius.
The *arbor philosophica* is growing out of him.

reference being to the figure of the coiled female serpent, the goddess Kundalini.[176] This double spiral consists of the two nadis, *ida* and *pingala*, meaning sun and moon, respectively, which together weave a figure-eight around the central *susumna* nadi. The *susumna* is the Kundalini herself in all her glory, alone as a widow,[177] like *muladhara*. We become the spiral as we wind these masculine and feminine energies together with our breath.

Kundalini starts in the roots, in the *muladhara*-sacral region and moves toward the "thousand-petaled lotus" *(sahasrara)* at the crown of the head. Paradoxically, we are born out of both poles of this central axis, from the womb of the eternal mother and from the seed of the divine father. The spiral, which has neither beginning nor end, always returns by winding on to its source. From its opposite pole, the source of energy is able to see and reflect on itself from afar, thereby becoming conscious of itself. In this way heaven and earth separated and engendered the light of consciousness. It is our function as human beings to act as a link between heaven and earth, between the divine and human worlds. One way we do this is through the practice of yoga, through uniting body with psyche in glorious harmony. The tree pose, among others, brings us in line with the world axis.

Figure 25 gives an excellent representation of the journey of the Kundalini. We should note that there are only six chakras pictured here compared to the normal seven, the number we usually think of as completing the chakra system. The seventh chakra does not, strictly speaking, belong to the system per se; rather it is the place where consciousness comes in on the transcendental level and, therefore, it is often included in the chakra system. The ancient texts stated that if the energy force has flowed freely and opened the blockages on its way, then the energy is free to leave from the crown of the head and unite with the divine. It seems as if this energy almost jumps off the crown of the head in the joy of union with the divine. There will always be a part of this energy, however, that remains in the body and forces the

---

[176] See also above, p. 105.

[177] *Hatha Yoga Pradipika: Light on Hatha Yoga*, chapt. 3, verse 110, p. 381.

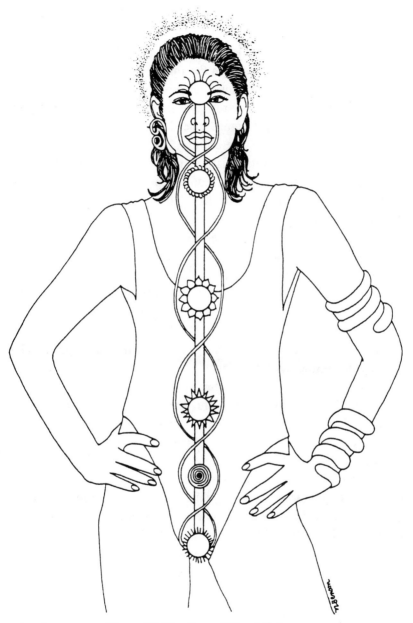

Figure 25. The flow of Kundalini energy.

descent once again, uniting with the chthonic world. It is only at the time of mortal death that all the energy leaves the body and goes through the veil to the other world.

We can also find the Kundalini in the image of the two serpents encircling the caduceus of Asclepius, our modern symbol for healing. Hans Holbein painted the popular image of two serpents with a dove sitting between them at the summit. The dove is placed there to balance out the strong power of the chthonic in the two encircling serpents (Figure 26). This painting is not unlike the alchemical picture discussed earlier, where an eagle is seen chained to a toad.[178]

Another typical portrayal of the Kundalini is with wings at the top of the ascent, symbolizing a "winged radiance" assumed to belong only to those who have achieved the delicate balance between the opposing forces of the two serpents (Figure 27). These wings are thought to be the lobes of the medulla, the petals of the third-eye chakra, whose vision of the union of body and soul has been realized through the practice.[179] In alchemy the soul evolves through the unfolding of two subtle energies, Sulphur and Quicksilver, conveying the notion of the two breaths of *ida* and *pingala* in the subtle body. Together they are termed Nature, hence it was repeatedly said: "Nature takes delight in Nature; Nature contains Nature; and Nature can overcome Nature."[180] These energies were thought to be the two serpents that encircled themselves around the caduceus, calling forth Mercurius, the healing power through which transformation took place (Figure 28).

As the Kundalini makes her double-spiraled ascent, she pierces each of the six chakras on her way, thus opening the energy along the spine. Each chakra is a center of energy that like all mandalas is a world unto itself. William Hauer defined the chakras as "symbols of the experience of life, they show the real inner meaning of such an experience, to help you to understand and to interpret spiritually what

---

[178] See above, p. 48.
[179] Jill Purce, *The Mystic Spiral*, p. 25.
[180] Quoted in ibid., p. 42.

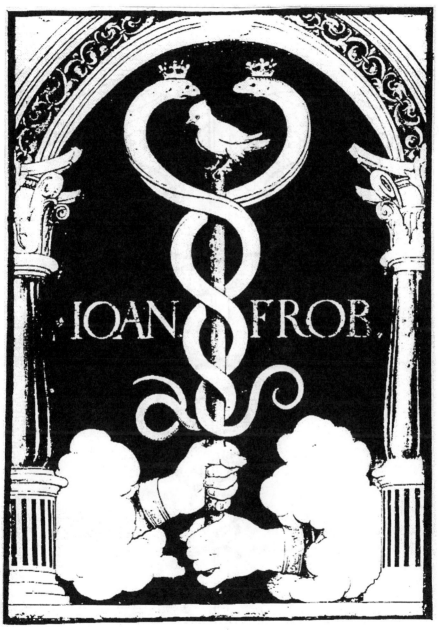

Figure 26. *Caduceus*, by Holbein, 1523.

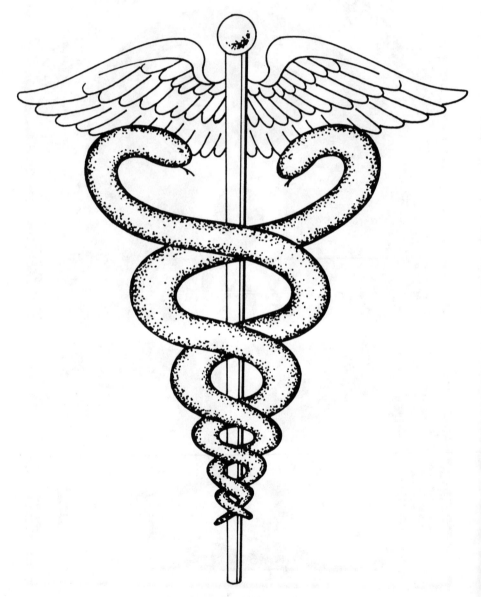

Figure 27. Caduceus.

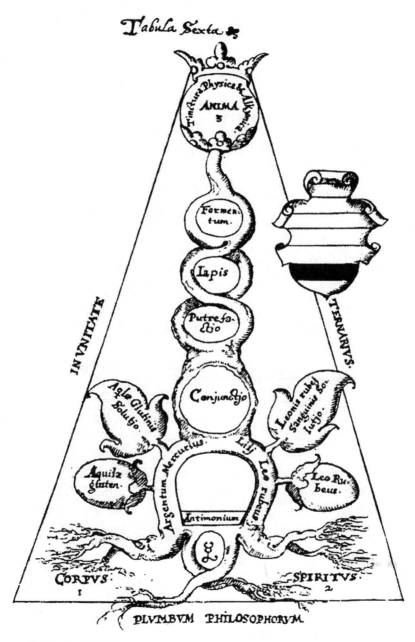

Figure 28. The evolution of the soul in the alchemical *magnum opus*.

you have lived."[181]

Light circles unremittingly in the eternal search for the center in each chakra. It is this process of circumambulation that brings us back to the original *prima materia*, the creative source within. Jung says:

> The potter's wheel rotates on the ground and produces earthenware ("earthly") vessels which may figuratively be called "human bodies." Being round, the wheel refers to the self and the creative activity in which it is manifest. The potter's wheel also symbolizes the recurrent theme of circulation.[182]

As if by a miracle, through the constellation of the *prima materia*, once the inner light has been discovered the entire chakra begins to rotate by itself. In *The Secret of the Golden Flower* it is said that the most important thing for achieving the circulation of the light is rhythmical breathing.[183] Positive light brings the embodiment of consciousness. As the focus of awareness becomes more and more concentrated, the center of each chakra becomes more distinct and more conscious, enabling us to relate to it in a clearer way. Each chakra has within itself the capability to develop a new part of the personality within an enclosed vessel, corresponding to its position on the spine. As the energy rises, consciousness intensifies.

Jung says that real consciousness only begins in *anahata*, the heart chakra,[184] which would mean that the lower chakras are unconscious. I do not agree with Jung on this point. Again I feel there is too much emphasis on the motif of ascension. People usually think of the chakra system as only an upward movement of energy toward the divine above. One may not want to be grounded; it may feel too uncomfortable to live in the reality of life. Too little has been said about what happens to the energy when it comes back down to earth. Gopi

---

[181] *Yoga, Especially the Meaning of the Chakras*, quoted in Jung, *The Psychology of Kundalini Yoga*, p. 3, n 2.

[182] "Individual Dream Symbolism in Relation to Alchemy," *Psychology and Alchemy*, CW 12, par. 281.

[183] Wilhelm, *The Secret of the Golden Flower*, p. 44.

[184] *The Visions Seminars*, p. 1232.

Krishna reported that his Kundalini energy traveled downward after its awakening.[185] Grounding in *muladhara* brings in a sense of awareness that brings the body to consciousness.

As the Kundalini mounts the spinal column touching each chakra as she travels, the energy is carried from one chakra to the next higher one, encompassing and absorbing that which is lower. Thus, when the Kundalini rises out of *muladhara* to the next chakra, *svadhisthana* (located at the level of the sexual organs and identified with water), the earth element becomes reabsorbed into, and encompassed by, the water element. Similarly, water is reabsorbed into fire at the next level, *manipura* (at the level of the navel); fire into air in the *anahata* chakra (at the level of the heart); and air into ether in the *visuddhi* chakra (located in the throat).[186]

Chakras are also called lotuses, symbolizing the unfolding of flower petals as each chakra is opened. The lotus flower is sacred in India and represents the development from the *prima materia* to the full light of consciousness, which, mirroring *muladhara*, unfolds into the thousand-petaled lotus at the crown. Chakras, like flowers, may be open or closed, blossoming or dying, depending on the state of consciousness within. It is said in the ancient texts that, as the Kundalini travels up the spinal column, she pierces and releases each lotus flower which then turns its head upward as she passes through. This would mean that there is always a correspondence between an upturned lotus and a down-turned one, except in *muladhara* before the serpent is aroused and in *sahasrara* before the beginning of the descent. It is important to realize that the entire ascent of the Kundalini serpent is against the normal downward flow of bodily fluids with gravity; it is this movement of energy against nature that grants yogic deliverance.

When the Kundalini energy has attained its goal and reached the crown, *sahasrara*, it does not simply remain there in its final resting point. There is instead a natural tendency of Kundalini to return to its source along with the flow of gravity. The energy remains in *sahas-*

---

[185] Judith Anodea, *Wheels of Life*, p. 68.
[186] White, *The Alchemical Body*, p. 208.

rara as long as the yogin is able to hold his or her concentration. In accordance with *enantiodromia*, however, there will always be a tendency for the energy to return to its original source, *muladhara*, the root of all life.

We must always keep in mind that when sufficient energy accumulates it will turn around and flow into its opposite. This process of reversal is necessary in order to avoid one-sidedness. The motif of descent follows the age-old ritualistic journey which leads down to the underworld where the dark night of the soul must be confronted in the quest for wholeness. During the ascent of light within the chakra system, there is an increase of consciousness. Similarly, during the descent, impurities are gradually liberated, allowing a cleansing and releasing that brings renewal each time. As the impurities are disposed of the whole process begins once again, but on a higher level which brings the renewal of consciousness. The mystics almost always pictured this descent in a spiral; the world was created by bringing heaven down to earth in the incarnation of matter uniting heaven and earth in *coniunctio*.

In various world traditions there is an image of an upside-down tree which, in yogic terms, mirrors the inverted poses such as headstand and shoulderstand. While holding the position of reversing gravity, a more stable relationship to the central spinal axis develops, bringing a sense of balanced well-being and energy both to the body and to the psyche. Inverted poses are wonderful for correcting imbalances as well as for restoring natural energy in times of depletion. They always help to bring a new perspective to a complex, often allowing one to quickly see a completely different point of view. This upside-down image is found in several representations of the inverted tree in the Upanishads, for example, as well as in this verse from the *Bhagavad Gita*:

> There is a fig tree
> In ancient story,
> The giant Ashvattha,
> The everlasting,
> Rooted in heaven,

Its branches earthward;
Each of its leaves
Is a song of the Vedas,
And he who knows it
Knows all the Vedas.

Downward and upward
Its branches bending
Are fed by the gunas,
The buds it puts forth
Are the things of the senses,
Roots it has also
Reaching downward
Into this world,
The roots of man's action.[187]

It is actually a reversal of attitude that is needed. In the *Hatha Yoga Pradipika*,[188] we learn that the benefits of the inverted poses have to do especially with reversing the flow of a specific fluid away from the brain center. Semen is transformed into ambrosia, the divine nectar of immortality, when the natural upright position of the body becomes reversed. The roots are then in the divine realm, allowing the fluids to flow back toward the head without strain (Figure 29), effecting total yogic integration, a reversal of time that evokes the immortal presence within us. Semen transforms into the nectar of immortality as it rises along the *susumna* nadi.

The main force behind the transformation of mundane semen (as it is called in Tantric alchemy) into the divine nectar of immortality and of the mundane mind to a state beyond mind is a pneumatic one. It is wind that provides the dynamic element which, in the form of disciplined breathing, plays the crucial transformative role in the system of hatha yoga. It is through *pranayama* (breath control) that the

---

[187]*The Song of God* (trans. Prabhamananda and Isherwood), quoted in "The Philosophical Tree," *Alchemical Studies*, CW 13, par. 412.

[188] The *Hatha Yoga Pradapika* was written in the Middle Ages and is concerned with physical exercises, breathing and cleansing techniques as ways of purifying the body on the road to transcendence.

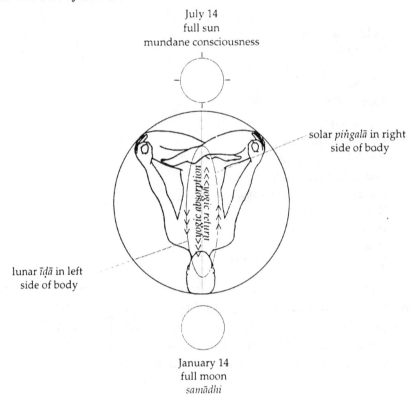

Figure 29. Yogic model of the year.

channels open for both the ascent and the descent of energies. Rather than purely descending, when the semen reverses the fluids are forced upward into the cranial vault where, held down by gravity, they unite in the *sahasrara* chakra with the divine in the transformation of the subtle body.

There is something of a prejudice in our culture toward the vertical approach to life, to the detriment of bodily reality. We must always remember that there are two world axes, the vertical representing spirit, perfection and the yearning for God, and the horizontal depicting the ego's relationship to reality through bodily experience. Renaissance painters emphasized the horizontal body and contact with the earth. This change brought with it an emphasis on the reality of daily life and the connection to Mother Earth. The emphasis on the horizontal came into being when people were beginning to come in contact with the reality of life and with the instinctual world. Matter, or mother, was the concern of this time. In contrast, the earlier Gothic period represented a longing for spiritualization, with the architecture consisting of elongated spirals that reached up toward the sky. As Jung wrote:

> It is as if the tremendous heights of the Gothic times were collapsing, sinking down to earth, and as if man were reaching *out*, instead of reaching *up* to heaven like the first fish. Energy was no longer heaped up, it extended horizontally; man then discovered the earth.[189]

Within the vast realm of bodywork available today, it is ironic that the horizontal realm is often overlooked. When we live in reality we are living in a body that naturally accepts, if given half a chance, its own height and breadth, which take their shape organically when the breath begins to flow consciously. Suddenly we experience living in a body that is able to rejoice in being alive. Trust develops out of the tiniest kernel of growth. Many of us, in unconsciously trying to be as small and inconspicuous as possible, have shortened and collapsed inward, not only in a vertical direction, but in width as well. Collapsing inward often has to do with terrible feelings of shame about who we are in the world. Such a posture serves only to cramp our breathing apparatus, not allowing us to be fully present in life, therefore not allowing us to utilize our full physical as well as creative potential. A great deal of energy is taken up in a huge effort to breathe, but in a completely unnatural way. The ribs must be free to expand and contract with the breath. The ribcage is not a rigid, inflexible structure as most of us have been taught, but rather a structure that relishes movement with each breath. In fact, respiration moves the many joints of the ribcage in a complex manner. Generally speaking, the upper ribs move up and down like a pump handle, whereas the lower ribs move up and down in a consistent circular motion. When our movements are limited, so are our possibilities for wholeness. We are meant by

---

[189] *The Visions Seminars*, p. 549.

nature to exist as a fourfold anatomical structure. As human beings we embody a greater totality through the union of the divine and human realms.

Simon, a young man of twenty-five, came to see me a few years ago complaining of a lack of direction in his life. Although he was a top student at university, he was not at all sure that, after graduation, he wanted to work in the field that he had been studying. Simon is a very tall and exceedingly thin man. Until recently he would often bring in dreams of creatures from outer space, smashed cars and so on, all images of an inability to be on this earth. His genetic body type had exaggerated the problem but, in addition, Simon had developed a very rigid upright stance that pulled him away from the earth, away from the force of gravity; thus he lacked flexibility, both mentally and physically. His rigidity drove him to put his ideas into very narrow boxes, stifling his creativity; and it was with this attitude that he lived his life.

As Simon was not rooted in *muladhara*, he suffered from severe prostatitis, an unusual symptom for a man in his mid-twenties. When I met him he had been so ill that he had developed an intolerance to antibiotics and was being forced to find another solution to the intense physical pain which often paralyzed him. Simon desperately yearned for a meaningful spiritual life that would be different from his upbringing as the son of a well-known minister in Germany. But without the grounding of the earth to hold him down, Simon was often almost literally flying away in the sessions with me. On a physical level, he was using only his muscles to keep himself upright rather than relying on the spine, the backbone of life. In the end he was left with no real support. In reality, Simon had very little sense of security about his body or from the inside where he suffered from feelings of inferiority with regard to his masculinity. His body had become sick in the prostate region, that is, at the level of masculinity in the root chakra.

In the beginning of the analysis, I tried each hour to pull him toward the earth, into reality. In fact his paintings invariably showed very little sky. At first this may seem misleading as one would expect his paintings to be dominated by the upper world in light of his constant yearning for spirit. But if we look behind this yearning, we see that he is actually possessed by matter, by the devouring feminine. Simon's yearning to grow upward, to leave life altogether, is an attempt to escape the devouring mother. The lack of sky in his paintings showed clearly his yearning for spirit, for a connection to the father archetype which would give him a stance against the devouring mother. Simon is possessed by a negative mother complex.

I have never done any bodywork with Simon, but in all our sessions I have been constantly aware of his body. His rigidity has considerably softened through a new-found ability to find expression for his feelings. A few months ago he brought in the following dream that he had after an hour of analysis:

> I see in the gymnasium at my school a spine that is constructed out of people. The people form each vertebra with their bodies. They are bound together through having their hands on the belly of the man or woman that is standing in front of them. The people have a huge ability of movement within this spinal structure that is at the same time very stable. There is a huge amount of trust as each person is holding on to the belly of the one in front. There is no eye contact, only body contact. The people are behind one another and all the trust comes from behind. This trust comes actually through touch.

This dream brought a compensating horizontal aspect to Simon's one-sided vertical standpoint in life. The beginnings of consciousness were surfacing. Simon had come into contact with the Platonic Original Round Man. I have also seen dreams where there seems to be a confusion between the horizontal and vertical approaches to life. Both sides must be held at once in the duality of psyche and matter. Within our own body we must never forget that what we are trying to achieve in the end is a conscious return to how we were prior to the creation of heaven and earth.

Coming back to Jung's notion that the serpent actually sleeps in the lumbar region, not in *muladhara*, as is generally thought, we find ourselves back to the number five, to the *quinta essentia*. Historically, five is particularly associated with ascension. David M. Knipe has shown that the number three illustrates the vertical cosmos envisioned in elevation, reaching up to the third and highest world (assuming the three worlds of heaven, earth and the underworld).[190] Four is the horizontal cosmos stretching to the four corners of the earth, and five is both at once and, therefore, the most complete expression of the world in its entirety. It then follows that the center pivotal point within the five is in correspondence with all three vertical worlds as well as with the four quarters of the earth, effecting the *quinta essentia*, being that it is all and everything.

Returning to the Midrashic legend that tells of angels moving up and down on Jacob himself and not on the ladder, we learn that Jacob becomes the focus of the angels' activity as they taunt him while he sleeps spread-eagled on the earth, held fast in the grip of gravity.[191] God gives him the ground on which he is lying.[192] Jacob embodies both the spiritual and physical aspects as he lies spread out on the ground dreaming of the angels ascending and descending on the axis between heaven and earth. The Bible tells us how Jacob prepared for the dream that was to change his life:

> And Ya'aqov went out from Be'er-sheva, and went toward Haran. And he lighted on a certain place, and tarried there all night, because the sun was set; and he took of the stones of that place, and put them under his head, and lay down in that place to sleep.[193]

In the same Midrash mentioned above we find the commentary that Jacob took not just one stone, but twelve, foreshadowing that he would become the father of the twelve tribes of Israel.[194] Twelve was a very important number in the alchemical laboratory as it signified the number of operations that were to be carried out in the process of transforming base metals into gold. The number twelve is also related to time as there are twelve months of the year and twelve signs of the Zodiac. Here the timing is absolutely precise: it is only on this par-

---

[190] "One Fire, Three Fires, Five Fires: Vedic Symbols in Transition," in *History of Religions*, vol. 12, no. 1, August 1972.
[191] Zornberg, *Genesis: The Beginnings of Desire*, pp. 191ff.
[192] Gen. 28:13.
[193] Gen. 28:10-11.
[194] Zornberg, *Genesis: The Beginnings of Desire*, p. 196.

ticular night that Jacob lies down and has his numinous dream, as already discussed.[195]

Again, in the Midrash, it is said that Jacob sets the stones around his head, not as a pillow under his head, as we read in Genesis. His head, therefore, becomes the center in the middle of the twelve-stone formation which unites all possibilities within himself. As Zornberg relates, there is a variation of the twelve stones motif to be found in Midrash Pirke Eliezer 35 that describes the stones as coming

> from the altar on which Isaac his father was bound. . . . And they all became one stone, to tell Jacob that they were all destined to become one nation in the land. . . . And in the morning, Jacob sat down to gather the stones together (and replace them on the altar); and he found them all one stone, and he set it up as a pillar. . . . What did God do? He stretched out His right foot and sank the stone deep into the earth, as one inserts a keystone into an arch. Therefore it is called *Even Shetiya*—the Foundation Stone of the world.[196]

In ancient Israel, this Foundation Stone was the first solid material to emerge from the waters of creation, it was the *prima materia* and upon this stone the Supreme Being created the universe. According to Jewish legend, it was this particular primordial rock on which Jacob slept, at the place he subsequently named Bethel, whose original name was *Luz*. We could say that as Jacob himself became the ladder, he also becomes the stone, uniting all elements within himself in the image of wholeness. Paradoxically, he also serves as the goal of his own transformation; he is the *lapis philosophorum* that unites bridegroom and bride. Jacob appropriates his physical strength from his brother Esau by mercurially deceiving him out of the blessing that is his birthright, dons his "new skin," and, upon seeing his beloved Rachel for the first time, rolls away the stone.[197] Jacob's encounter with his anima was recounted in the Midrash when he takes the crucial step in leaving the home of his father:

---

[195] Above, p. 94.
[196] *Genesis: The Beginnings of Desire*, p. 198.
[197] Gen. 29:10.

When Jacob left his father's presence, he left adorned like a bridegroom and like a bride in her ornaments. And there descended on him reviving dew from heaven, and his bones were covered with fat; and he, too, became a champion fighter and athlete. That is why it is said: "By the hands of the Mighty One of Jacob—There, the shepherd, the rock of Israel." (Genesis 49:24)[198]

It is only after his numinous dream that Jacob was able to gather his strength and unite the masculine and feminine in holy matrimony. Metaphorically, the first man was made of the earth; the second as the redeemed came from heaven. Jacob, in uniting all aspects, manifests the completed world, as does Mercurius, and serves as mediator between the divine and the human. The necessity for the relatedness between these two worlds is explained by Jung:

> The beginning is divine and the end is divine, and between the two is the human being, the more earthly and the more heavenly being.[199]

The union of all and everything in Plato's Original Round Man resonates in subtle body. One of Jung's patients who had no previous knowledge of yoga drew an image (Figure 30) of the awakening of the Kundalini energy. We see how she has been able to envision the spiraling feminine energy that emerges out of the vessel created through the concentration of energy.

Flexible yet unshakable, we receive the love from the transcendent. The sun and moon unite in the *susumna* nadi as the breath brings golden light into the sacrum, taking us back to an earlier time and thrusting forward to the beginnings of a future era where creation occurs within the vessel of a conscious body.

---

[198] *Pirke d'Rabbi Eliezer*, 32, quoted in Zornberg, *Genesis, The Beginnings of Desire*, p. 178.
[199] *The Visions Seminars*, p. 294.

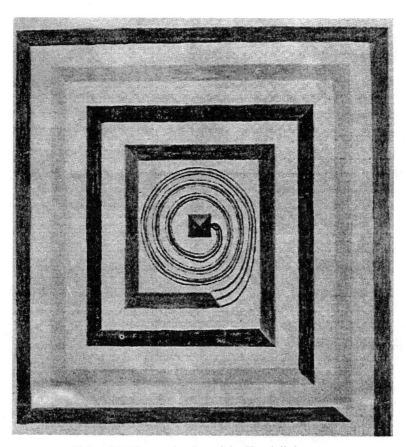

Figure 30. The awakening of the Kundalini energy.

Bibliography

Afterman, Allen. *Kabbala and Consciousness*. Riverdale-on-Hudson, NY: Sheep Meadow Press, 1992.

Anodea, Judith. *Wheels of Life*. St. Paul, MN: Llewellyn Publications, 1987.

Avalon, Arthur. *The Serpent Power*. New York: Dover Publications, 1974.

ben Shimon Halevi, Z'ev. *Adam and the Kabbalistic Tree*. Bath, UK: Gateway Books, 1985.

_____. *The Way of Kabbala*. Bath, UK: Gateway Books, 1976.

Birkhäuser-Oeri, Sibylle: *The Mother: Archetypal Image in Fairy Tales*. Toronto: Inner City Books, 1988.

Budge, E.A. Wallis. *The Gods of the Egyptians*. Mineola, NY: Dover, 1969.

Campbell, Joseph. *The Mythic Image*. New York: MJF Books, 1974.

Cirlot, J.E. *A Dictionary of Symbols*. New York: Dorset Press, 1971.

Cook, Roger. *The Tree of Life*. London, UK: Thames and Hudson, 1974.

Desikachar, T.K.V. *The Heart of Yoga*. Rochester, VT: Inner Traditions International, 1995.

Dowd, Irene. *Taking Root to Fly*. New York: Contact Collaborations, 1981.

Edinger, Edward F. *The Creation of Consciousness: Jung's Myth for Modern Man*. Toronto: Inner City Books, 1984.

_____. *The Mysterium Lectures: A Journey through Jung's* Mysterium Conunctionis. Toronto: Inner City Books, 1995.

Eliade, Mircea: *The Forge and the Crucible: The Origins and Structures of Alchemy*. Chicago: University of Chicago Press, 1978.

_____. *Images and Symbols*. Princeton: Princeton University Press, 1991.

_____. *Patterns in Comparative Religion*. Lincoln, NB: University of Nebraska Press, 1958.

_____. *Shamanism: Archaic Techniques of Ecstasy* (Bollingen Series LXXVI), Princeton: Princeton University Press, 1964.

_____. *Yoga: Immortality and Freedom* (Bollingen Series LVI). Princeton: Princeton University Press, 1958.

Epstein, Perle. *Kabbala: The Way of the Jewish Mystic*. Boston: Shambhala, 1988.

Feuerstein, Georg. *Yoga: The Technology of Ecstasy.* Los Angeles: Jeremy P. Tarcher, 1989.

Finkel, Avraham Yaakov. *In My Flesh I See God.* London, UK: Jason Aronson, 1995.

Franklin, Eric. *Dynamic Alignment Through Imagery.* Champaign, IL: Human Kinetics, 1996.

Frazer, James G. *The Golden Bough.* Abridged ed. London: Papermac, 1987.

Ginzberg, Louis. *Legends of the Bible.* Philadelphia: The Jewish Publication Society, 1956.

Gosh, Schyam. *The Original Yoga.* New Delhi: Munschiram Manoharlal Publishers, Ltd., n.d.

Gottlieb, Freema. *The Lamp of God.* London, UK: Jason Aronson, 1989.

Graves, Robert. *The Greek Myths.* Middlesex, UK: Penguin Books, 1955.

Harding, M. Esther. *Psychic Energy: Its Source and Goal.* Washington, DC: Pantheon Books, 1947.

Hardy, Friedhelm. *The Religious Culture of India.* Cambridge, UK: Cambridge University Press, 1994.

Hatha Yoga Pradipika. Munger, Bihar, India: Bihar School of India, 1993.

Heschel, Abraham Joshua. *God in Search of Man: A Philosophy of Judaism.* New York: Farrar, Straus and Giroux, 1955.

Howey, M. Oldfield, *The Encircled Serpent.* New York: Arthur Richmond Company, 1955.

The I Ching or Book of Changes (Bollingen Series XIX). Trans. Richard Wilhelm. Princeton: Princeton University Press, 1967.

Isler, Gotthilf. "The Kiss of the Snake." Unpublished paper.

Jerusalem Bible. Jerusalem: Koren Publishers, 1992.

In The Image of Man: The Indian Perception of the Universe through 2000 Years of Painting and Sculpture. Hayward Gallery, London, 1982. London: The Arts Council of Great Britain, 1982.

Jung, C.G. *The Collected Works* (Bollingen Series XX), 20 vols. Trans. R.F.C. Hull. Ed. H. Read, M. Fordham, G. Adler, Wm. McGuire. Princeton: Princeton University Press, 1953-1979.

_____. *Letters* (Bollingen Series XCV). 2 vols. Ed. G. Adler. Princeton: Princeton University Press, 1973-1975.

_____. *Modern Psychology: Notes on Lectures Given at the Eidgenössische Technische Hochschule, Zurich, 1938-40.* Zurich: C.G. Jung Institute, 1959.

_____. *Nietzsche's* Zarasthustra (Bollingen Series XCIX). 2 vols. Ed. James L. Jarrett. Princeton: Princeton University Press, 1988.

_____. *The Psychology of Kundalini Yoga* (Bollingen Series XCIX). Princeton: Princeton University Press, 1996.

_____. *The Visions Seminars* (Bollingen Series XCIX). Ed. Claire Douglas. Princeton: Princeton University Press, 1997.

Jung, Emma, and von Franz, Marie-Louise: *The Grail Legend.* Boston: Sigo Press, 1986.

Knipe, David M. "One Fire, Three Fires, Five Fires: Vedic Symbols in Transition." In *History of Religions*, vol. 12, no. 1 (August 1972).

Kohn, Livia. *Taoist Meditation and Longevity Techniques.* Ann Arbor, MI: Center For Chinese Studies, 1989.

Krishna, Gopi. *Living with Kundalini.* Boston: Shambhala, 1993.

Kushner, Lawrence. *The River of Light.* San Francisco: Harper and Row, 1981.

Leeming, David Adams, and Leeming, Margaret Adams. *A Dictionary of Creation Myths.* Oxford: Oxford University Press, 1994.

Lindsay, Jack. *The Origins of Alchemy in Graeco-Roman Egypt.* London, UK: Frederick Muller, 1970.

Lundquist, John M. *The Temple: Meeting Place of Heaven and Earth.* London, UK: Thames and Hudson, 1993.

Maguire, Anne. *Hauterkrankungen als Botschaft der Seele* (The Fire and the Serpent). Olten, Germany: Walter-Verlag, 1991.

Murche, Guy. *The Seven Mysteries of Life.* Boston: Houghton Mifflin, 1978.

Myers, Esther. *Yoga and You.* Toronto: Random House, 1996.

Myers, E., and Echlin, K. "Awakening the Spine." In *Yoga Journal*, June 1966.

Myers, Esther, and Lynn Wylie. *The Ground, the Breath, & the Spine.* Toronto: Self-published, 1990.

Patai, Raphael. *The Jewish Alchemists.* Princeton: Princeton University Press, 1994.

Perera, Sylvia Brinton. *Descent to the Goddess: A Way of Initiation for Women.* Toronto: Inner City Books, 1981.

Purce, Jill. *The Mystic Spiral: Journey of the Soul.* London, UK: Thames and Hudson, 1974.

Radha, Swami Sivananda. *Hatha Yoga: The Hidden Language.* Spokane, WA: Timeless Books, 1995.

Radhakrishnan, Sarvepalli, and Moore, Charles A., eds. *A Sourcebook in Indian Philosophy.* Princeton: Princeton University Press, 1957.

Sansonese, J. Nigro. *The Body of Myth.* Rochester, VT: Inner Traditions International, 1994.

Scaravelli, Vanda. *Awakening The Spine.* London, UK: Aquarian Press, 1991.

Scholem, Gershom. *The Messianic Idea in Judaism.* New York: Schocken Books, 1971.

Seton-Williams, M.V. *Egyptian Legends and Stories.* London, UK: The Rubicon Press, 1988.

Stewart, Mary. *Yoga.* London, UK: Hodder and Stoughton, 1992.

Tansley, David V. *Subtle Body: Essence and Shadow.* London, UK: Thames and Hudson, 1977.

Kohn, Livia, ed. *Taoist Meditation and Longevity Techniques.* Ann Arbor, MI: Center For Chinese Studies, 1989.

Todd, Mabel E. *The Thinking Body.* Princeton: Princeton Book Company, 1937.

Unterman, Alan. *Dictionary of Jewish Lore and Legend.* London, UK: Thames and Hudson, 1991.

The Upanishads. Trans. Eknath Easwaran. Tomales, CA: Nilgiri Press, 1987.

von Durkheim, Karlfried Graf. *Hara: The Vital Center of Man.* London, UK: Mandala Books, 1977.

von Franz, Marie-Louise. *Alchemy: An Introduction to the Symbolism and the Psychology.* Toronto: Inner City Books, 1980.

_____. *Aurora Consurgens.* 2nd ed. Toronto: Inner City Books, 2000.

_____. *Creation Myths.* Revised ed. Boston: Shambhala, 1995.

_____. *The Feminine in Fairy Tales.* Dallas: Spring Publications, 1972.

_____. *The Interpretation of Fairy Tales.* Boston: Shambhala, 1996.

_____. *Number and Time.* Evanston, IL: Northwestern University Press, 1979.

_____. *On Dreams and Death*. Boston: Shambhala, 1987.

_____. *The Psychological Meaning of Redemption Motifs in Fairy Tales*. Toronto: Inner City Books, 1980.

Westman, Heinz. *The Springs of Creativity*. Wilmette, IL: Chiron, 1986.

White, David Gordon. *The Alchemical Body*. Chicago: University of Chicago Press, 1996.

Wilhelm, Richard, trans. *The Secret of the Golden Flower*. New York: Harcourt Brace Jovanovich, 1962.

Woodman, Marion. *Addiction to Perfection: The Still Unravished Bride*. Toronto: Inner City Books, 1982.

_____. *Conscious Femininity: Interviews with Marion Woodman*. Toronto: Inner City Books, 1993.

_____. *The Ravaged Bridegroom: Masculinity in Women*. Toronto: Inner City Books, 1990.

Woodman, Marion, and Dickson, Elinor. *Dancing in the Flames*. Toronto: Alfred A. Knopf, 1996.

Zimmer, Heinrich. *Myths and Symbols in Indian Art and Civilization* (Bollingen Series VI). Princeton: Princeton University Press, 1972.

Zornberg, Avivah Gottlieb. *Genesis: The Beginnings of Desire*. Philadelphia: Jewish Publication Society, 1995.

Index